Atlas of Male Infertility Microsurgery

Marc Goldstein

Atlas of Male Infertility Microsurgery

Springer

Marc Goldstein
Center for Male Reproductive Medicine and Surgery
Weill Cornell Medicine
New York-Presbyterian Hospital
New York, NY, USA

ISBN 978-3-031-31600-5 ISBN 978-3-031-31601-2 (eBook)
https://doi.org/10.1007/978-3-031-31601-2

This Springer imprint is published by the registered company Springer Nature Switzerland AG
The registered company address is: Gewerbestrasse 11, 6330 Cham, Switzerland

To all my fellows, residents, and students from whom I have learned as much as I have taught.

To my wife Barbara, without whose encouragement and support this Atlas would never have happened.

Preface

My interest in microsurgery began when my father gave me a 1920's vintage brass monocular microscope that he had used at The City College of New York. The world inside a droplet of standing water on the sidewalk in front of our family house provided hours of fascination. In medical school, I did stereotaxic neurosurgery, inserting penicillin crystals in the lateral geniculate body of cats to induce secondary epileptogenic foci.

After graduating *summa cum laude* from the College of Medicine, State University of New York—Downstate Medical, I did my internship and residency in general surgery at Columbia Presbyterian Medical Center in New York. At the time, the Vietnam War was still raging, and I took time off from residency to go into the Air Force and become a rated Flight Surgeon, training at the School of Aerospace Medicine. I was one of the lucky few who got assigned to a tactical reconnaissance squadron where I flew as a flight surgeon in F-4 Phantom (RF-4C) for 3 years (Fig. 1). Instead of guns, we had cameras. I flew between 50 and 500 feet at 500 knots and took pictures. Appropriate to my profession, I never killed anyone. I jokingly tell patients now that the hand-eye coordination involved in doing microsurgery is very similar to the hand-eye coordination involved in flying high-performance aircraft. The biggest difference is: back then it was my butt on the line, and now it's their balls.

After my military service, I did my urology training at SUNY Downstate Medical Center in the late 1970s. At that time, operating microscopes were unknown to the field. One day, I saw an article by Italian microsurgeons who had surgically transplanted a testicle from one man to

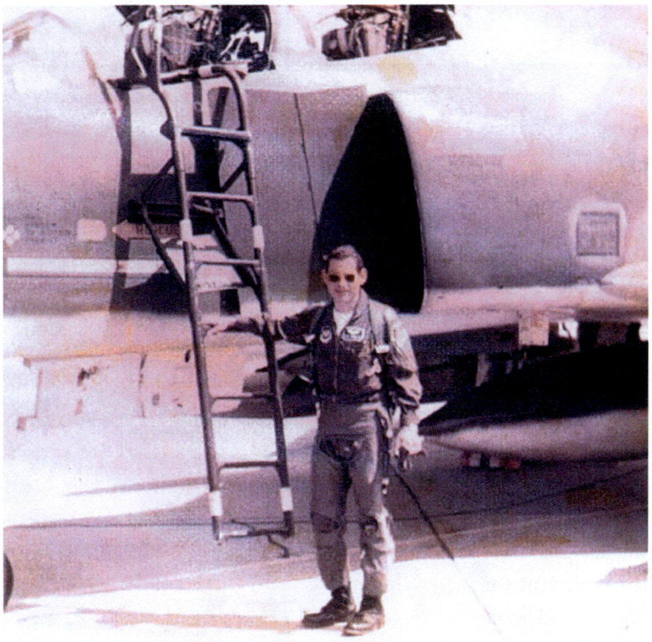

Fig. 1 Dr. Marc Goldstein standing with his F-4 Phantom (RF-4C)

his identical twin who had lost both testicles. The recipient of the transplant fathered a child with his brother's testicle. The transplant required anastomosis of the tiny testicular artery, testicular vein, and vas deferens. Simultaneously, Dr. Sherman Silber reported an identical case in the United States. Around the same time, Dr. Earl Owen, in Australia, and Silber, his former fellow, reported successful reanastomosis of the vas deferens for vasectomy reversal. My Chairman, Dr. Keith Waterhouse, sent me to Saint Louis to learn from Silber the only urologic microsurgeon in the world at that time.

I came back from that visit with Dr. Silber intent on making a career in urologic microsurgery. The only microscope in the hospital was in neurosurgery, and I practiced microsurgery in the closet where the microscope was kept, using pieces of fresh human placenta to practice vascular anastomosis. This resulted in my first publication [1].

When I finished my urology residency, there were no training programs in microsurgery, or male reproductive urology, so I went to Rockefeller University to work with an endocrinologist, the late great C. Wayne Bardin, MD who was interested in this area. I suggested to him that I wanted to transplant testicles in rats. Could we use that as a model for understanding how the hypothalamic-pituitary-testis axis works? He thought it was a great idea, but no one had ever successfully transplanted testicles in rats with microsurgery. So, I developed the technique myself. I was given an operating microscope and was able to operate on rats (Fig. 2). For around 6 months, I could not get a single transplant to work. However, as I learned how to do the microsurgery better and better, I slowly started to see success. Each transplant of a rat testicle took all day. Sometimes, I would lose animals to anesthesia, so I learned how to resusci-

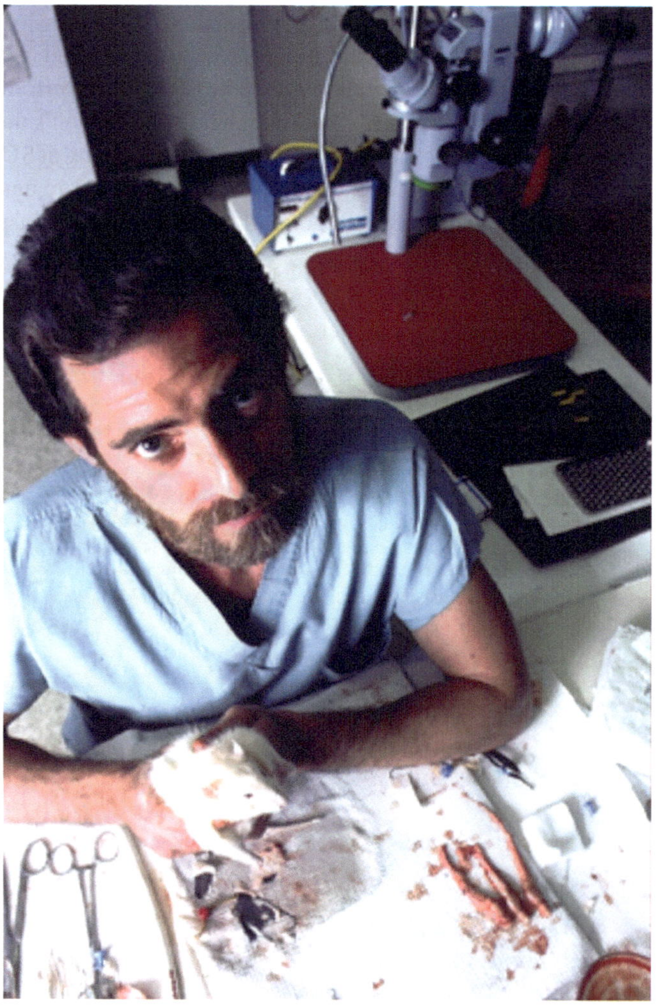

Fig. 2 Dr. Marc Goldstein with a rat during his fellowship at Rockefeller University

tate them by putting a tube in my mouth and the other end of the tube in the rat's mouth. It was the head of my laboratory, the late Kalyan Sundaram, PhD who was watching me do this and he asked me how I knew which end of the tube belonged to me and which end belonged to the rat. This question led to his major contribution to my research: he labeled one end of my tube "Marc" and the other end "Rat."

It quickly became apparent that there was a tremendous need for a specialist in my area, and that this need was unmet and we therefore needed to develop training programs. I started the first fellowship program around the same time as Larry Lipschultz at Baylor, and the rest is history.

I edited my first book *Surgery of Male Infertility* in 1995 [2], in which I solo-authored half of the chapters. While the ones I didn't write were excellent, I would have done those a bit differently and, I thought, better.

Years later, I stumbled onto Shlomo Raz's classic *Atlas of Transvaginal Surgery* [3] which, I am told by the publishers, has been the best-selling book in urology for 20 years. Shlomo, is considered the master in his field. He trained several of our Cornell Urology residents who later developed reputations as outstanding surgeons. I, rather unhumbly, consider myself the "Shlomo Raz" of my field. I always dreamed of writing a book like his, where every word, every photograph, every video is done by me.

In this Atlas, you should imagine you are my fellow, assisting me in the operating room.

References/Recommended Reading

1. Goldstein M. Use of fresh human placenta for microsurgical training. J Microsurg 1979;1:70–1.
2. Goldstein M. (ed.) Surgery of male infertility. Saunders; 1995.
3. Raz S. Atlas of transvaginal surgery. Saunders; 2002.

New York, NY, USA Marc Goldstein

Acknowledgments

To:

Vanessa L. Dudley, MSHS, true co-author of this atlas, a brilliant medical illustrator who did all the drawings and reviewed hundreds of photos and videos, choosing the best ones to use. Also it was able to transcribe my handwritten scrawl with which I wrote the entire atlas.

Dianis Rivera, who helped transcribe my scrawl and administered my practice so competently, allowing Vanessa time to work on the Atlas.

Philip Shihua Li, MD, Director of our Microsurgical Laboratory and Training Program who created the first laboratory of its kind, trained dozens of our residents, fellows, and visitors, and developed the animal models on which most of the innovations described in this Atlas are based.

Miriam Feliciano, who, in addition to helping Dr. Li run the Microsurgery Laboratory, performed the semen analyses on which our assessment of the efficacy of the procedures described herein are based.

Peter N. Schlegel, MD, who, in 20 years as Chair of Urology, helped train dozens of residents and fellows, many of whom have gone on to become Chairs at major institutions. In describing my best fellows, I always say "best since Schlegel." Peter also first authored the Male Infertility Guidelines of both the American Urological Association and the American Society of Reproductive Medicine in which many of the procedures described in this Atlas are recommended as the preferred methods.

Richard K. Lee, MD, MBA, Director of Residency Training, who has contributed to our resident training and research in such a major way and directed residents with interest and/or need to our Microsurgery Laboratory.

Finally, to my late, great mentors, R. Keith Waterhouse, MD, C. Wayne Bardin, MD, and E. Darracott Vaughan, MD.

To Zev Rosenwaks, MD, classmate, collaborator and friend for almost 60 years who has enthusiastically supported my sometimes radical ideas and work.

Contents

1 Microsurgical Training

Microsurgery is important in male infertility because of the microscopic size of the testicular vessels and ducts that are involved in sperm transport. The epididymis is approximately 15 ft. long but fits into a structure about the size of your pinky. The diameter of the epididymal tubule is about 150 μm in diameter; for reference, one of the hairs on your head is 100 μm in diameter. The outside diameter of the vas deferens is about 2 mm, but the tiny opening the sperm goes through is 300 μm, three times the diameter of a hair on your head. The testicular artery, the main blood supply to the testis, is 1–1.5 mm in diameter.

Many studies have shown that microsurgery is by far the best technique for fixing obstruction of the vas or epididymis. The most common cause of male infertility is varicocele, which is responsible for 35% of all cases of male infertility, 70% if you were once fertile and have since become infertile (secondary infertility). Because varicocele causes a progressive decline in fertility over time if it is not treated, varicocelectomy, if properly performed, will, at the least, preserve, and in a majority of men, enhance testicular function. The most common complications from doing this without an operating microscope are much lower chances of the surgery actually working, a significant incidence of testicular atrophy and worsening testicular function and, in 10% of men, development of a hydrocele, requiring a second operation. Using an operating microscope allows preservation of the 1.5 mm diameter testicular artery, preservation of lymphatics to prevent hydrocele, and the ability to identify and ligate all spermatic veins. Our research on the over 5000 patients on whom I have performed this surgery has clearly shown that you can virtually eliminate the risk of hydrocele (I have had none in the last 3500 cases) and reduce varicocelectomy failure rates to less than 1%, as well as prevent ligation of testicular artery causing the testicle to atrophy.

Almost all of the procedures described in this book are performed using an operating microscope. Competent use of the operating microscope requires training, and this should not be learned on patients. Ideally, this training should be performed in a laboratory. Those who wish to specialize in this field should take a 1–2-year fellowship after completing their residency. In lieu of that, there are microsurgical training courses, similar to the one we provide at Weill Cornell Medicine under the direction of Dr. Philip Li, director of the microsurgical training program. Students are taught how to place microsutures, first on a training pad, then using silicone tubing which simulates the vas deferens for procedures such as vasovasostomy. Finally, procedures are carried out on live rats, including vasovasostomy, vasoepididymostomy, and even vascular anastomoses.

Microsurgical training can also be acquired by taking courses at the Annual Meetings of the American Urological Association, or at the American Society for Reproductive Medicine. However, nothing is a substitute for hands on training in a laboratory. The ability to use an operating microscope for microsurgical varicocelectomy takes a minimum of 10–20 h of microsurgical training. To become reasonably competent at finding the arteries and tying off all veins, typically 50–100 cases need to be performed before a surgeon can be considered competent. Ideally, this should be done during residency training. If you are interested in the field and you don't have microsurgical training available to you, then you should arrange for your Chairperson to send you to an institution for several months, or at the very least to take an intensive microsurgical training course.

The key principle here is that microsurgical training is essential before attempting the microsurgical procedures described in this book. Some of these procedures do not require substantial microsurgical training, such as the use of an operating microscope for better visualization during hydrocelectomy or during inguinal hernia repair to minimize the risk of injury to the vas deferens. But use of the operating microscope for varicocelectomy, vasovasostomy, and vasoepididymostomy requires significant training (Figs. 1.1 and 1.2).

M. Goldstein, *Atlas of Male Infertility Microsurgery*, https://doi.org/10.1007/978-3-031-31601-2_1

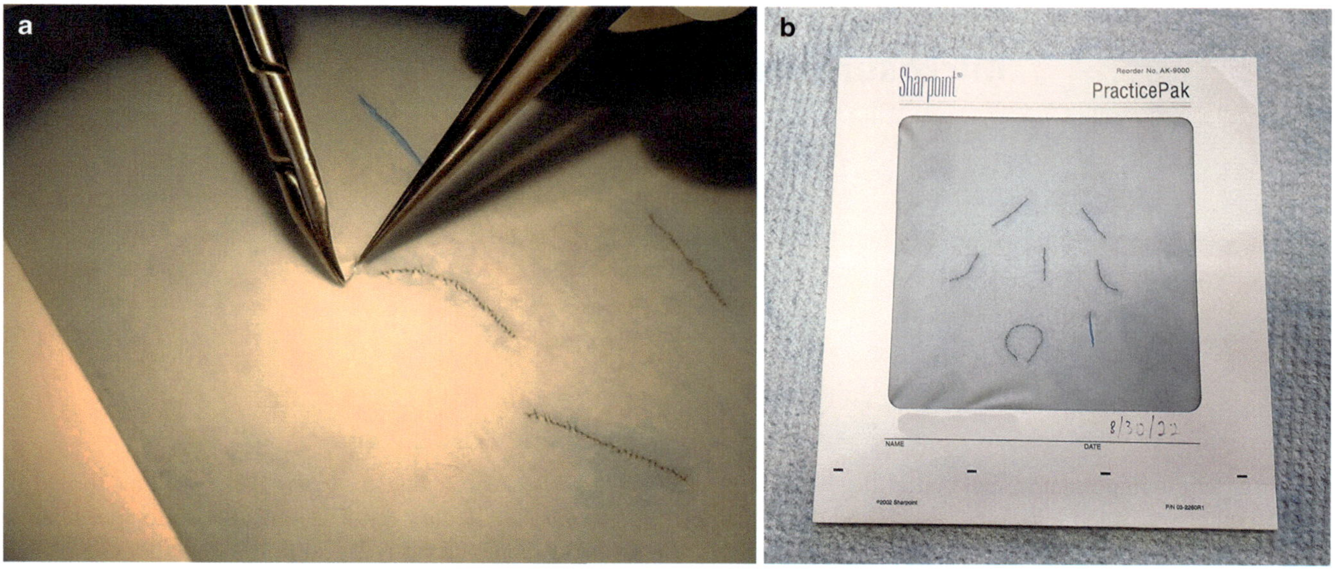

Fig. 1.1 (**a, b**) Students are taught how to place microsutures on a training pad first

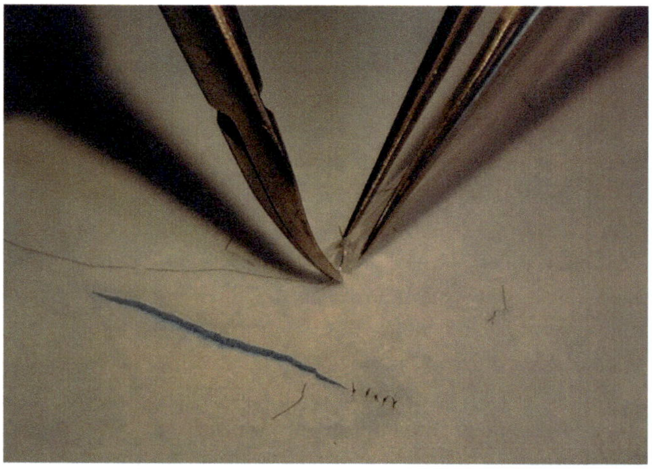

Fig. 1.2 Students are taught to use silicone tubing to simulate vasovasostomy

Anatomy of the Male Reproductive System

2

2.1 Introduction

A clear understanding of the anatomy of the male reproductive tract is essential to planning and carrying out these procedures.

2.2 Landmarks

Cutaneous landmarks allow employment of the perfect incision which ultimately saves time by providing the best exposure (Fig. 2.1a, b). Subcutaneous landmarks include

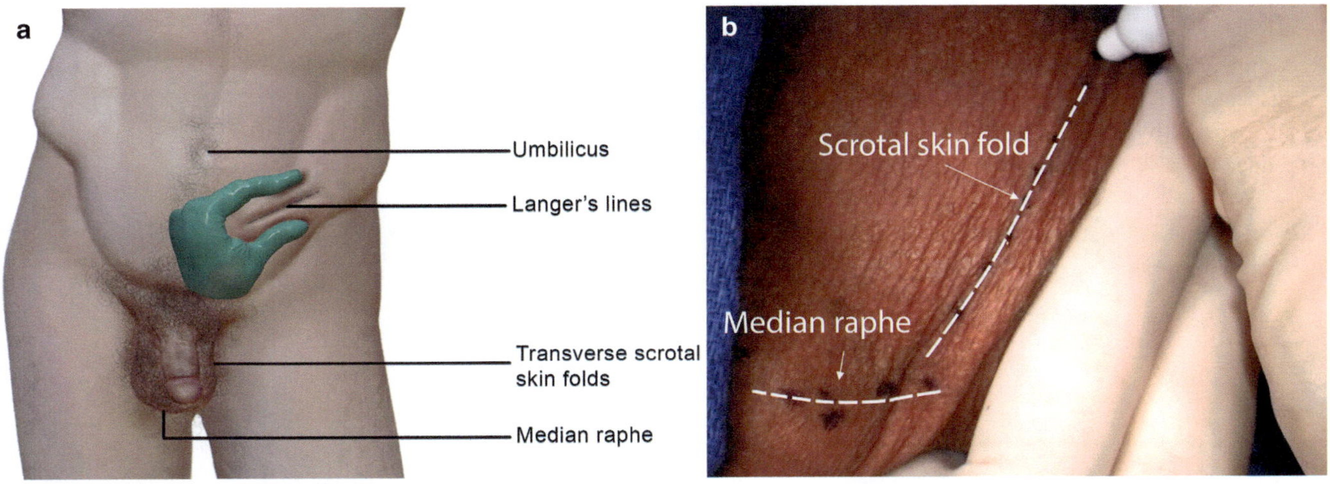

Fig. 2.1 (**a** and **b**) Cutaneous landmarks

M. Goldstein, *Atlas of Male Infertility Microsurgery*, https://doi.org/10.1007/978-3-031-31601-2_2

the anterior superior iliac crest, the femoral artery, the external inguinal ring, and the pubic tubercle (Fig. 2.2). Invagination of the relaxed scrotum with the index or ring finger just over the pubic bone allows identification of the underlying external inguinal ring, from which the spermatic cord exits (Fig. 2.3). Putting an "X" on the skin at ½ or 1 cm inferior to the external inguinal ring so the cord makes a gentle curve instead of a right angle helps prevent compression of the testicular artery against the external inguinal ring (Fig. 2.4).

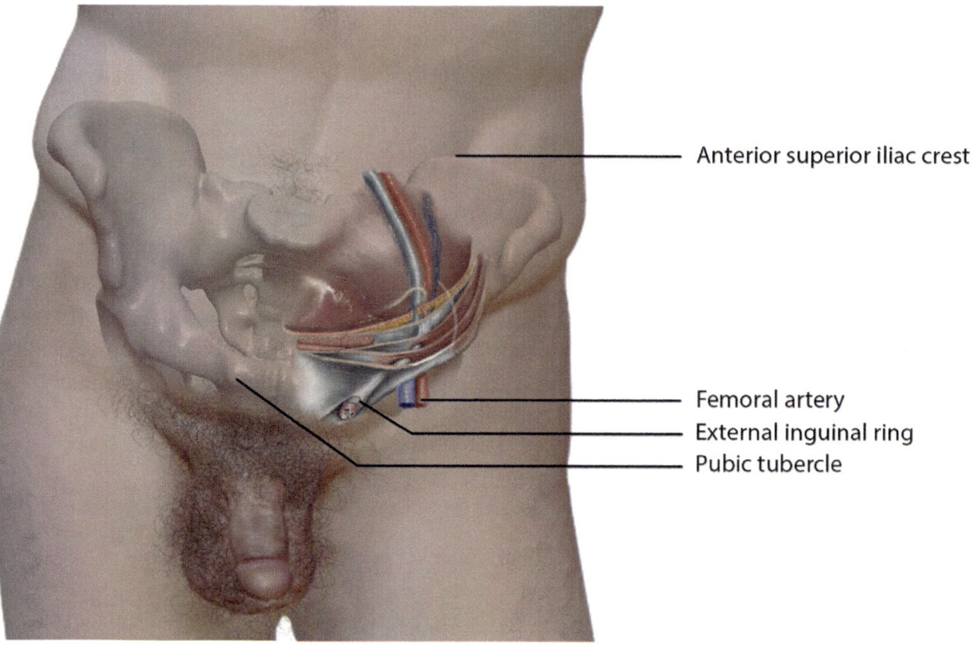

Fig. 2.2 Subcutaneous landmarks

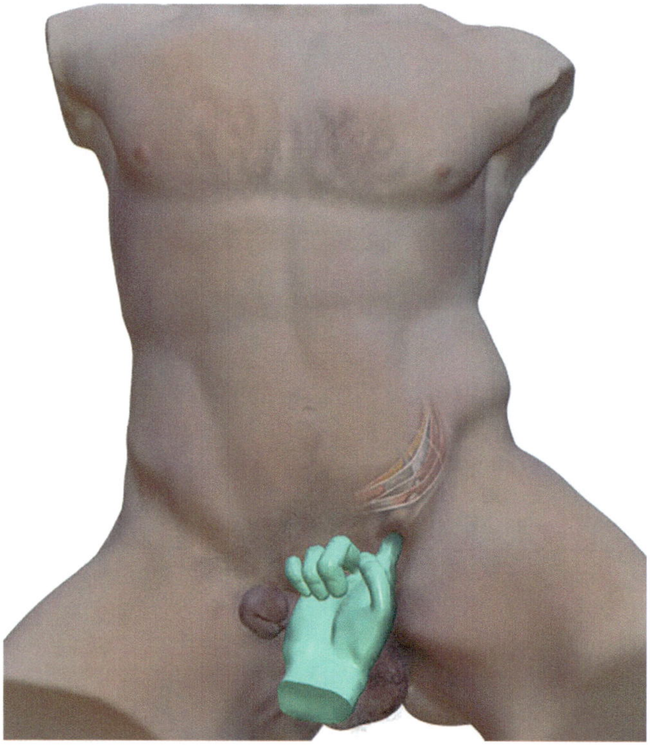

Fig. 2.3 Invagination of the relaxed scrotum with the index finger just over the pubic tubercle bone

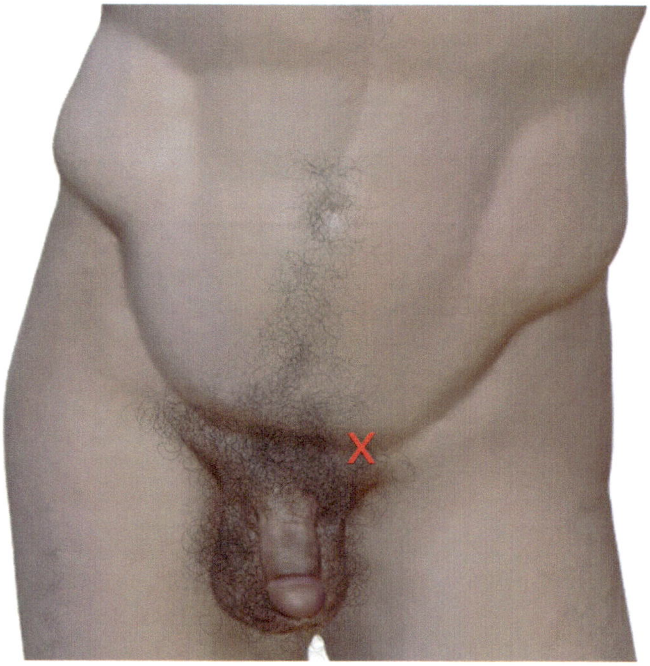

Fig. 2.4 An "X" on the skin ½ or 1 cm inferior to the external inguinal ring so the cord makes a gentle curve instead of a right angle. This helps prevent compression of the testicular artery against the external inguinal ring

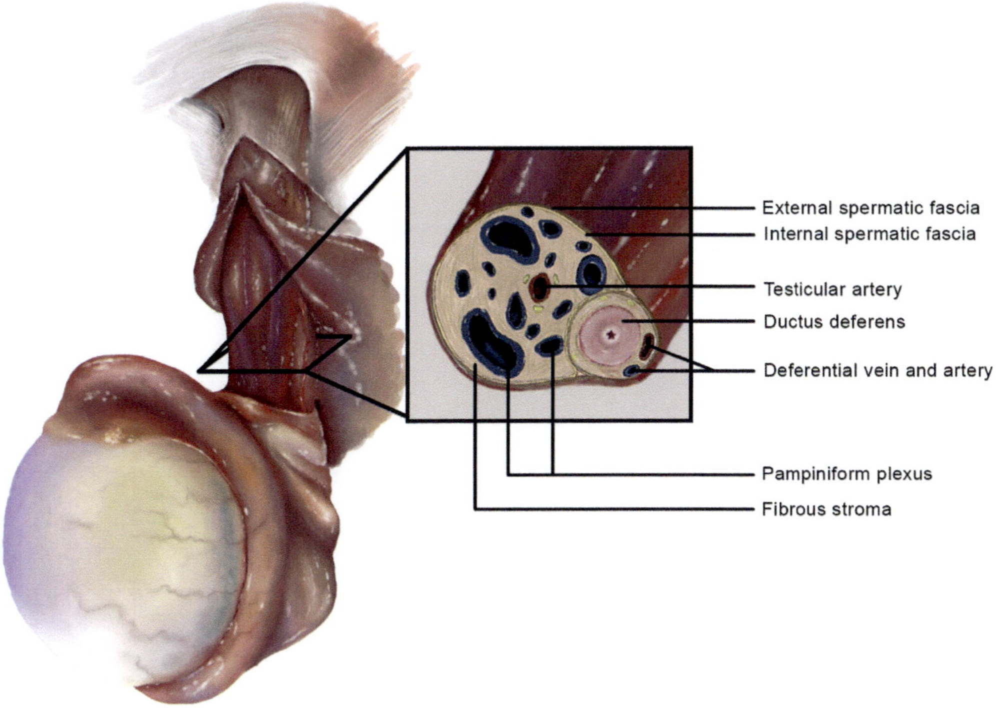

Fig. 2.5 The relationship between the vas deferens, the spermatic vessels, and spermatic fascia

2.3 Anatomy of the Spermatic Cord

The relationship between the vas deferens, the spermatic vessels, and spermatic fascia is shown in Fig. 2.5. Note that the internal spermatic fascia surrounds the internal spermatic vessels, but not the vas, which is found between the internal and external spermatic fascias, usually in the posterior lateral aspect of the cord.

Suggested Reading

Goldstein M. Surgical management of male infertility. In: Partin AW, Dmochowski RR, Kavoussi LR, Peters CA, Wein AJ, editors. *Campbell Walsh Wein Urology*. 12th ed. Amsterdam: Elsevier; 2020. Chapter 67.

Goldstein M, Mehta A. Male reproductive system. In: Standring S, editor. Gray's anatomy. 41st ed. London: Elsevier; 2015. p. 76.

Hopps CV, Lemer ML, Schlegel PN, Goldstein M. Intraoperative varicocele anatomy: a microscopic study of the inguinal versus subinguinal approach. J Urol. 2003;170:2366–70.

3 Microsurgical Subinguinal Varicocelectomy

Varicocelectomy is the most common fertility procedure performed in men. The most satisfying ones have huge varicoceles. When it goes away post-op, the patients are thrilled, and the outcomes are so good because the bigger the varicocele the bigger the improvement after successful repair.

3.1 Procedure Description

The procedure can be performed inguinally or subinguinally. If subinguinal, the incision is made along Langer's lines, over the external ring, and is approximately 2.5–3.5 cm in length (smaller incisions for small, atrophic testes and larger incisions for larger testes) (Fig. 3.1). After making the skin incision with a 15 blade, just deep enough so that the white subcutaneous layer and a bit of the "little" fat of Camper's fascia shows, the Bovie electrocautery, set at low cutting, is used to deepen the incision to the "big fat globules" layer (Fig. 3.2). A clamp is introduced anterior to Scarpa's fascia and with the hand beneath the Crile, the remainder of Camper's is divided using the Bovie on the cautery setting. The hand is always placed between the instrument and skin to prevent a Bovie burn if the instrument is accidentally touched by the Bovie (Fig. 3.3).

The superficial epigastric artery and vein at the superior aspect of the wound and/or the superficial external pudendal artery and vein at the inferior aspect of the wound, if encountered, are double clamped with curved mosquito clamps, divided, and ligated with 3-0 Vicryl. The clamp is pushed past the superior and inferior aspects of the skin wound and dragged back, dividing the remaining Scarpa's fascia, providing maximum exposure through the smallest incision. The left index finger is then hooked under the external inguinal ring, and a small Richardson retractor is placed on the back of that index finger and gently pulled, revealing the cord, usually identified by the large veins seen through its sheath (Fig. 3.4). The cord is grasped with the Babcock

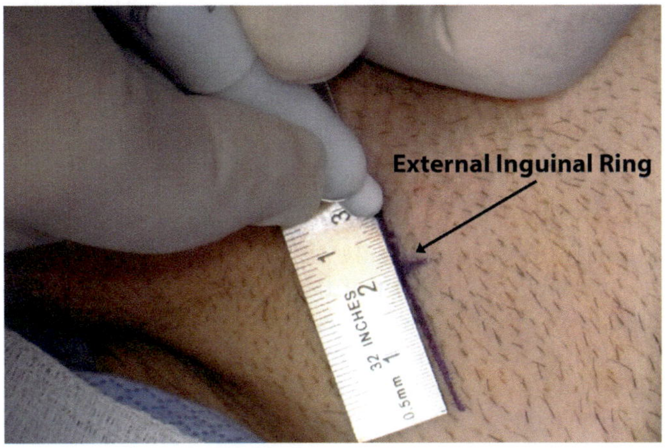

Fig. 3.1 The procedure can be performed inguinally or subinguinally. If subinguinal, the incision is made along Langer's lines, over the external ring, and is approximately 2.5–3.5 cm in length (smaller incisions for small, atrophic testes and larger incisions for larger testes)

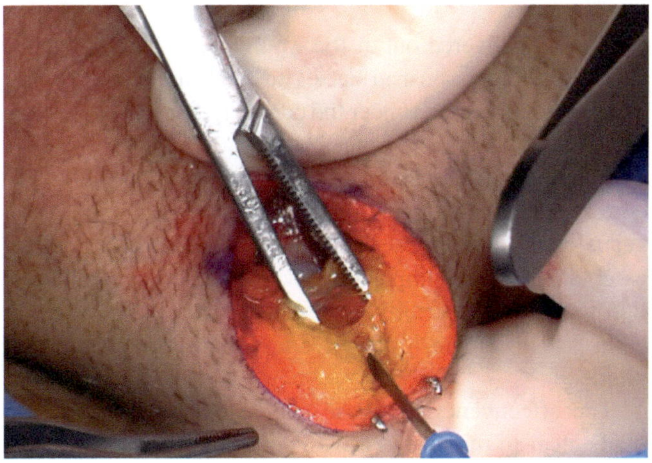

Fig. 3.2 After making the skin incision, the Bovie electrocautery, set at low cutting, is used to deepen the incision to the "big fat globules" layer

Supplementary Information The online version contains supplementary material available at https://doi.org/10.1007/978-3-031-31601-2_3.

M. Goldstein, *Atlas of Male Infertility Microsurgery*, https://doi.org/10.1007/978-3-031-31601-2_3

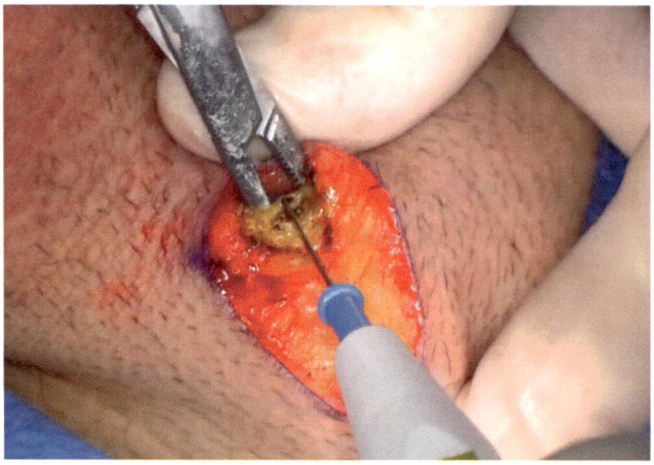

Fig. 3.3 A clamp is introduced anterior to Scarpa's fascia and with the hand beneath the Crile, the remainder of Camper's is divided using the Bovie on the cautery setting

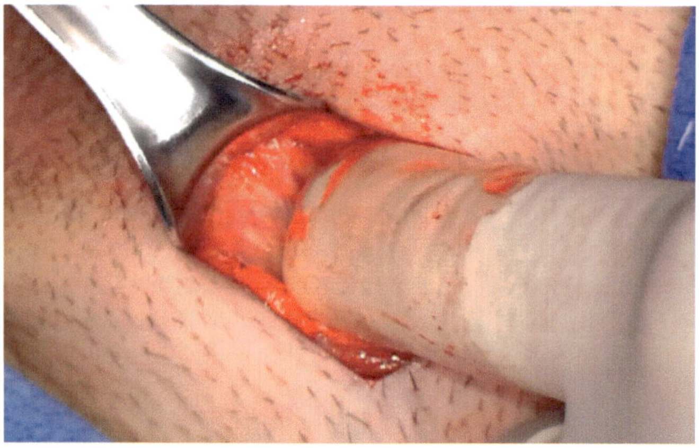

Fig. 3.4 The clamp is pushed past the superior and inferior aspects of the skin wound and dragged back, dividing the remaining Scarpa's fascia, providing maximum exposure through the smallest incision. The left index finger is then hooked under the external inguinal ring, and a small Richardson retractor is placed on the back of that index finger and gently pulled, revealing the cord, usually identified by the large veins seen through its sheath

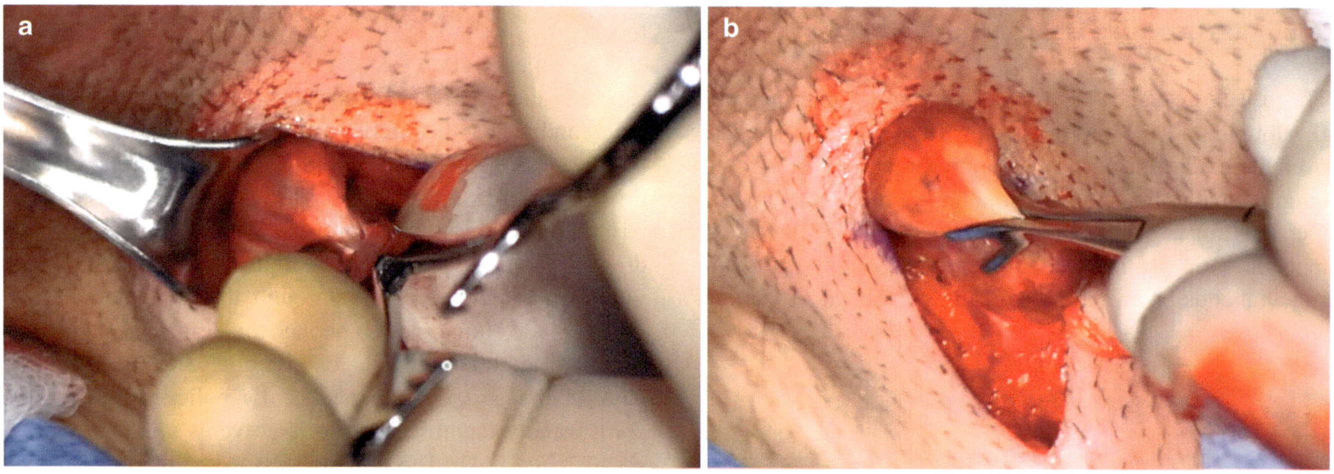

Fig. 3.5 (**a, b**) The cord is grasped with the Babcock clamp and delivered out of the wound

clamp and delivered out of the wound (Fig. 3.5a, b). Using two index fingers pushed back and forth under the cord, a clean opening is made under the cord (Fig. 3.6) and a medium Penrose drain is placed beneath it (Fig. 3.7a–c).

The operating microscope is brought into the field. The cord is pulled down by pulling on the testis as the index finger is gently manipulated around the cord and through the external ring. This simple maneuver allows the microdissection to start as superiorly as possible where there are fewer veins and the main testicular artery is less likely to have divided.

The effectiveness of these simple maneuvers has been made clear to me when I have gone back to repair inguinal hernias in men on whom I had previously performed subinguinal varicocelectomy. Upon opening the external oblique to perform a microsurgically assisted inguinal hernia repair (see Chap. 13), I noted that the micro-clips indicating the location of my prior varicocelectomy are in the mid-inguinal canal, almost as cephalad as when performing my original microsurgical inguinal varicocelectomy [1]. The time and effort in getting more cephalad on the cord is more than made up for by an easier microsurgical varicocelectomy.

Under 6–10× magnification, the external spermatic fascia is divided in the direction of its fibers with the Bovie (Fig. 3.8). The cephalad apex of this opening is identified, grasped with a small straight hemostat and a 5-0 vicryl suture on a small, tapered needle is placed at the apex and tied (Fig. 3.9). One end is left long and tagged with a small,

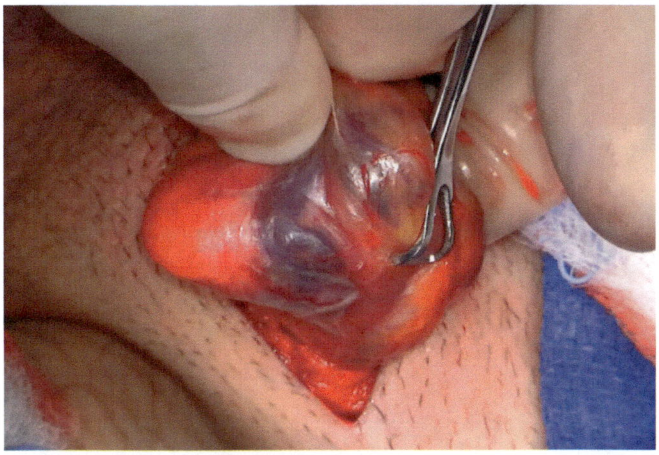

Fig. 3.6 Using two index fingers pushed back and forth under the cord, a clean opening is made under the cord

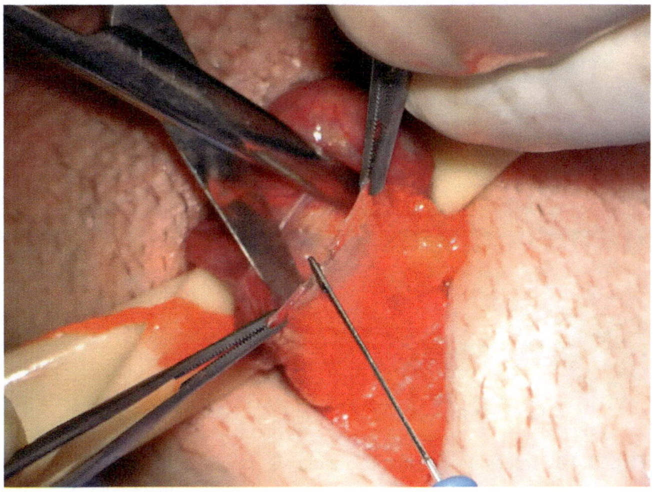

Fig. 3.8 External spermatic fascia is divided in the direction of its fibers with the Bovie

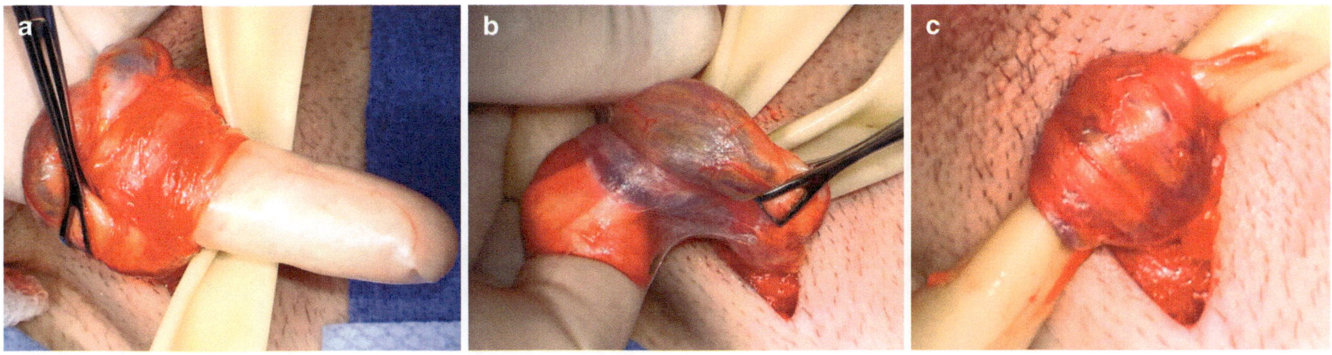

Fig. 3.7 (**a–c**) A medium Penrose drain is placed beneath the cord

curved hemostat. When the microdissection is complete, the suture is grasped, facilitating closure of the spermatic fascia. This covers the exposed arteries and restores the cord to as normal a state as possible. Interrupted sutures are used. You do not want a water-tight closure. If there is bleeding in the cord, better it come out around the cord than tamponade it (see later in this chapter).

Under 15× magnification, the internal spermatic fascia is opened with small, blunt scissors (Fig. 3.10). The bipolar cautery is used to control small vessels before cutting them. Never use the Bovie for the internal spermatic fascia, which is clear, thin, and relatively avascular. The testicular artery could be immediately subjacent and can be easily injured by the Bovie. The internal spermatic fascia is held open with four small hemostats, sequentially moved higher and higher on the cord (Fig. 3.11).

Under 15–25× magnification, a search is made for pulsations. A micro-Doppler is indispensable for certain identifi-

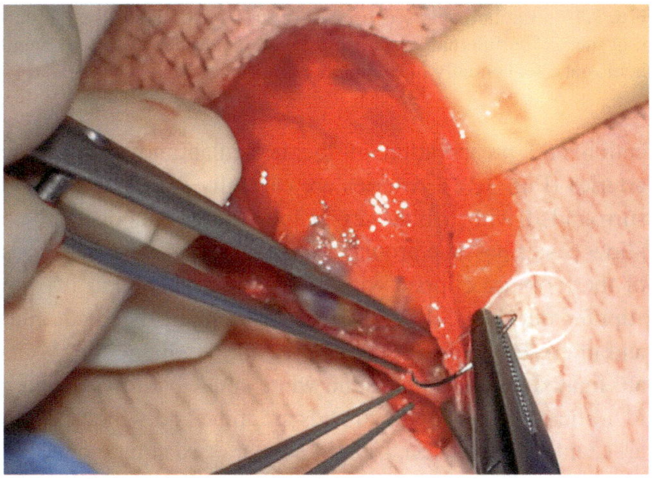

Fig. 3.9 The cephalad apex of this opening is identified, grasped with a small straight hemostat and a 5-0 vicryl suture on a small, tapered needle is placed at the apex and tied

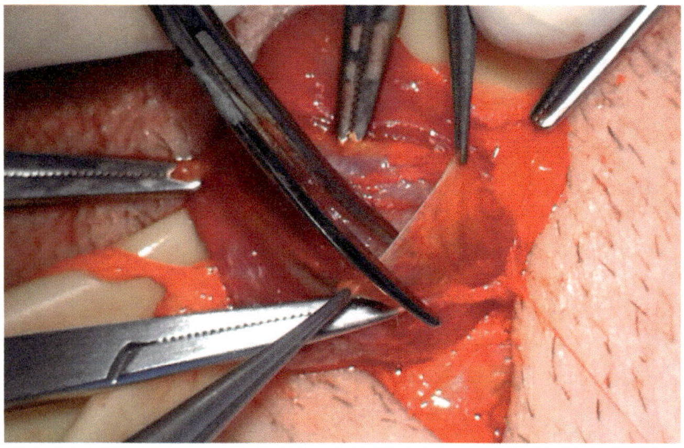

Fig. 3.10 Internal spermatic fascia is opened with small, blunt scissors

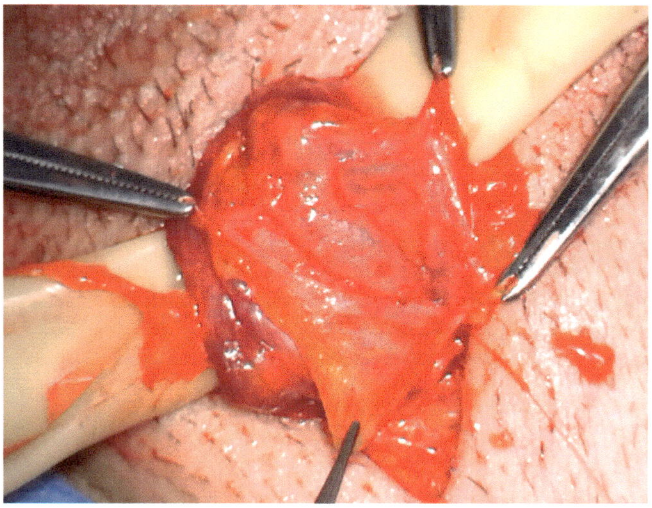

Fig. 3.11 Bipolar cautery is used to control small vessels before cutting them. The internal spermatic fascia is held open with four small hemostats, sequentially moved higher and higher on the cord

cation and preservation of the testicular and cremasteric arteries (Fig. 3.12). Arteries are carefully dissected out and surrounded with a blue vessel loop tapered at one end to allow easier passage around the artery (Fig. 3.13). The ends of the loop are clipped with a large clip to prevent it from slipping out (Fig. 3.14). A blunt, curved micro-needle holder and micro-toothed forceps are used for the dissection. Veins are ligated with 4-0 black and white sutures, allowing quick identification of which two ends are mine and which are the assistant's. (Fig. 3.15a, b) All knots are tied square and flat. Two square knots suffice for silk sutures only. Away from the arteries, veins are clipped and divided; I do not like a lot of metal around arteries.

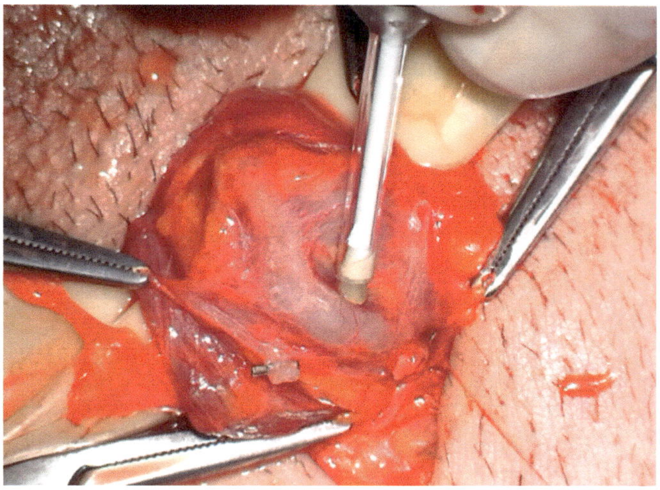

Fig. 3.12 Micro-Doppler is indispensable for certain identification and preservation of the testicular and cremasteric arteries

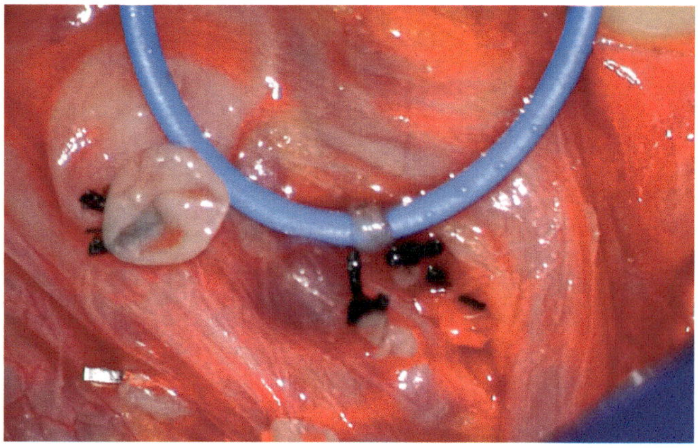

Fig. 3.13 Arteries are carefully dissected out and surrounded with a blue vessel loop tapered at one end to allow easier passage around the artery

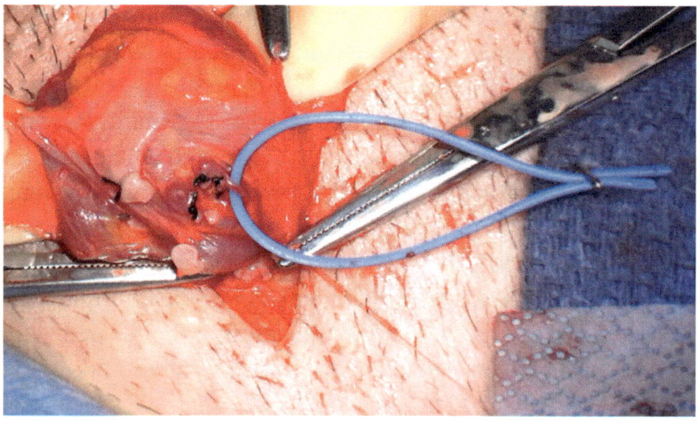

Fig. 3.14 Loop ends clipped with a large clip to prevent slipping out

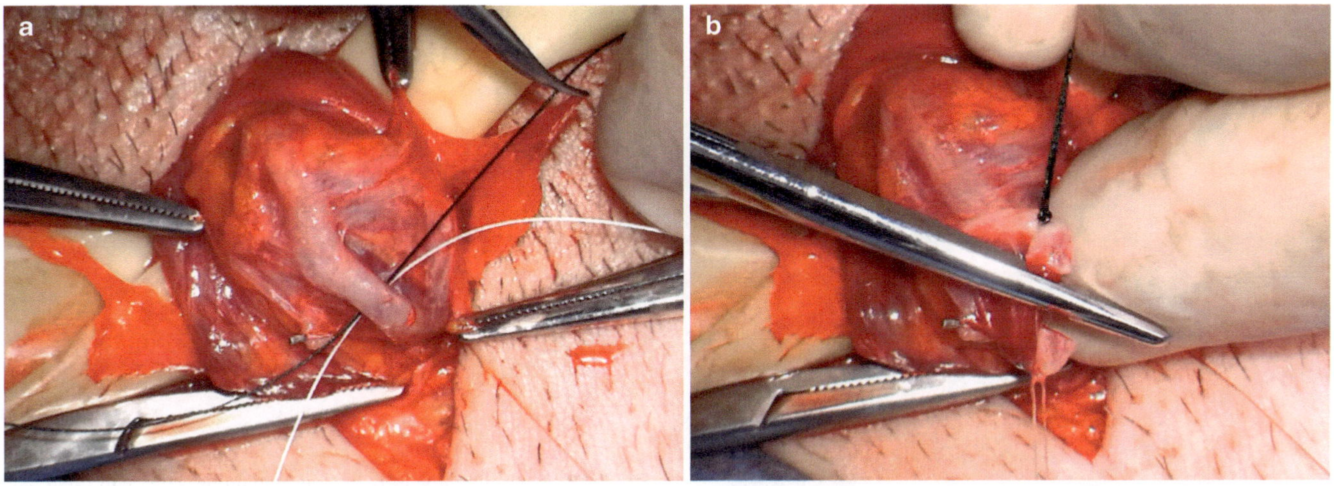

Fig. 3.15 (**a, b**) A blunt, curved micro-needle holder and micro-toothed forceps used for the dissection. Veins ligated with 4-0 black and white sutures to identify surgeon and assistant's ends

3.2 Partial Occlusion Test

Once putative arteries are identified with the operating microscope and micro-Doppler, absolute confirmation of the arterial nature of the vessel is made using what I call the partial occlusion test. Using the micro-needle holder placed under the putative artery, supported by the left index finger, the vessel is completely occluded with gentle upward pressure. The needle holder is slowly dropped down until a pulsating flash within the vessel has confirmed its arterial nature (Fig. 3.16; Video 3.1). A vessel loop is then placed around it and the loop clipped (see video). Arteries must have no veins stuck to them. These venae comitantes connect with large veins and can dilate up and cause a recurrence (Fig. 3.17).

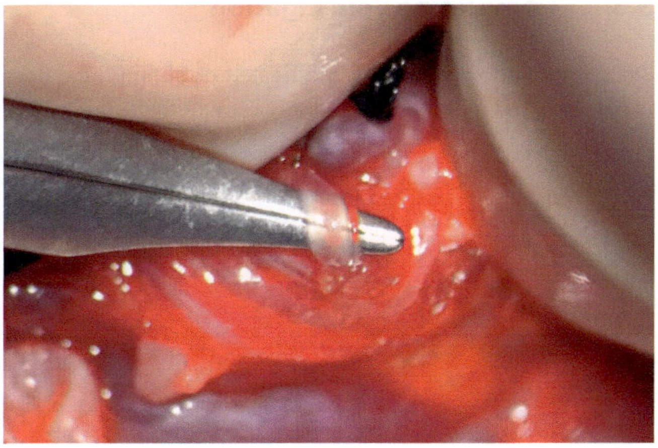

Fig. 3.16 Using the micro-needle holder placed under the putative artery, supported by the left index finger, the vessel is completely occluded with gentle upward pressure. The needle holder is slowly dropped down until a pulsating flash within the vessel has confirmed its arterial nature (see Video 3.1)

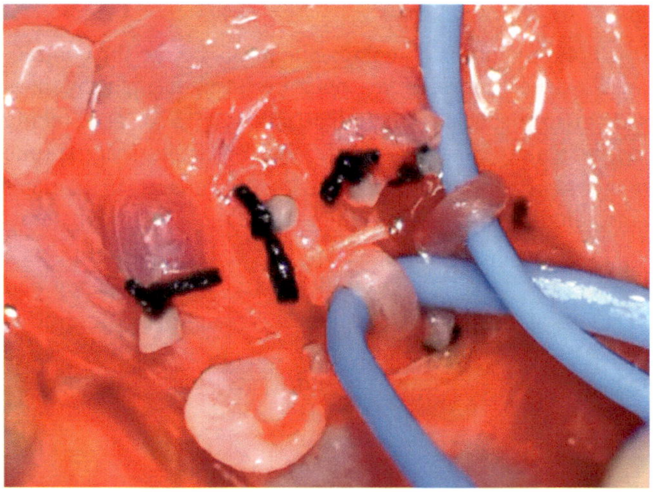

Fig. 3.17 A vessel loop is then placed around it and the loop clipped

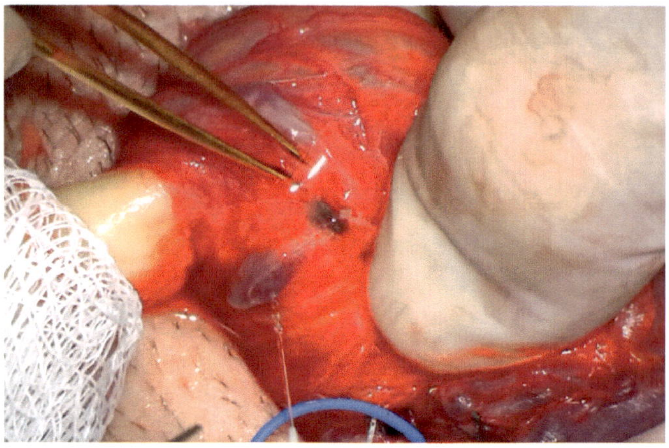

Fig. 3.18 Each time a vein is ligated, remaining veins will dilate and become more visible

3.3 Completing Vein Ligation

Once all major visible veins are ligated or clipped, the cord is run over the index finger and any remaining veins ligated or clipped. Each time a vein is ligated, any remaining veins will dilate and become more visible (Fig. 3.18). You must have one complete run through the cord without finding a single vein before you stop.

3.4 Vasal Veins

Abnormally dilated vasal veins can be a cause of failure, especially in children and adolescents [2]. After ligating the internal and external spermatic veins, the vas is inspected. The vas, as noted in Chap. 2, is not within the internal spermatic fascia, but between the internal and external spermatic facias (see Fig. 2.5). The vas is exposed and if a vasal vein is larger than 2.5 mm is found, especially if it is straight and not tortuous, as normal vasal veins are, it is ligated with 4-0 silk and divided. Prior to ligating a putative abnormal vasal vein, check with the micro-Doppler to make sure it is not a large vasal artery. If the abnormal vasal vein is ligated, rerun the cord to make sure the veins within the internal spermatic fascia have not become dilated.

3.5 Delivery of the Testis

Delivery of the testis is the only way to have direct visualization of every possible route of venous return (Fig. 3.19) [3]. Dr. Patrick Walsh, prior to inventing the nerve-sparing radical prostatectomy, was a fertility specialist, and even co-authored a book called *Male Infertility* [4]. He performed venograms on a series of failed surgical varicocelectomies and clearly demonstrated that 10% of failures were due to scrotal collaterals.

With the left hand, gently pulling on the cord, taking care not to pull on the vessel loops surrounding the arteries, and mostly pushing up on the testes with the middle and index fingers of the right hand, the testis is delivered (Fig. 3.20). Any external spermatic veins not running into the Penrose around the cord (these veins have already been ligated) are ligated and divided. A small Richardson retractor is placed in the lower aspect of the wound, exposing the gubernaculum. This is thinned out with two fingers until the edge of the tunica vaginalis is clearly seen (Fig. 3.21). Only veins exiting the tunica vaginalis and going into the scrotum are ligated. Once this is done, the tunica vaginalis is inspected for the presence of a hydrocele. More than 3 mL of hydrocele fluid can negatively impact testicular temperature regulation [5].

If a hydrocele is present, a wedge window excision is performed and the edges of the window cauterized with the Bovie, taking care to be far away from the epididymis (see Chap. 4) [5].

The testis is returned to the scrotum and the cord run again to make sure no additional veins have appeared. The spermatic fascia is reapproximated with interrupted sutures of 5-0 vicryl, pulling up on the suture placed at the apex when the spermatic fascia was initially opened (Fig. 3.22). I close the spermatic fascia because I don't like isolated arteries flapping in the breeze; I like putting things back as close to normal as possible. I use interrupted sutures because if there is bleeding from the site of ligation, I would rather go outside the cord instead of tamponading it. If there is still oozing at the ligation area, despite best efforts with the bipolar micro-cautery, Floseal is placed in the ligation area. Rarely, in redo varicocelectomies, I will place a Penrose drain in the dependent portion of the hemi-scrotum, fixed in place with a 2-0 silk stitch and a safety pin. This typically remains in place for 24–48 h postoperatively.

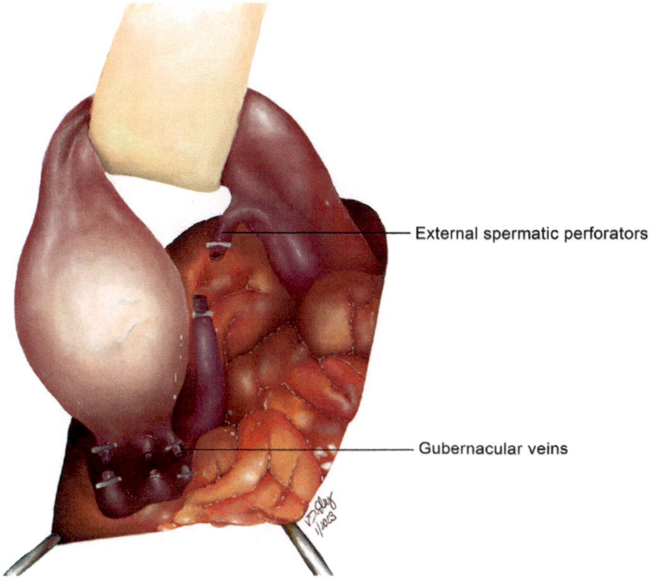

Fig. 3.19 Delivery of the testis is the only way to have direct visualization of every possible route of venous return

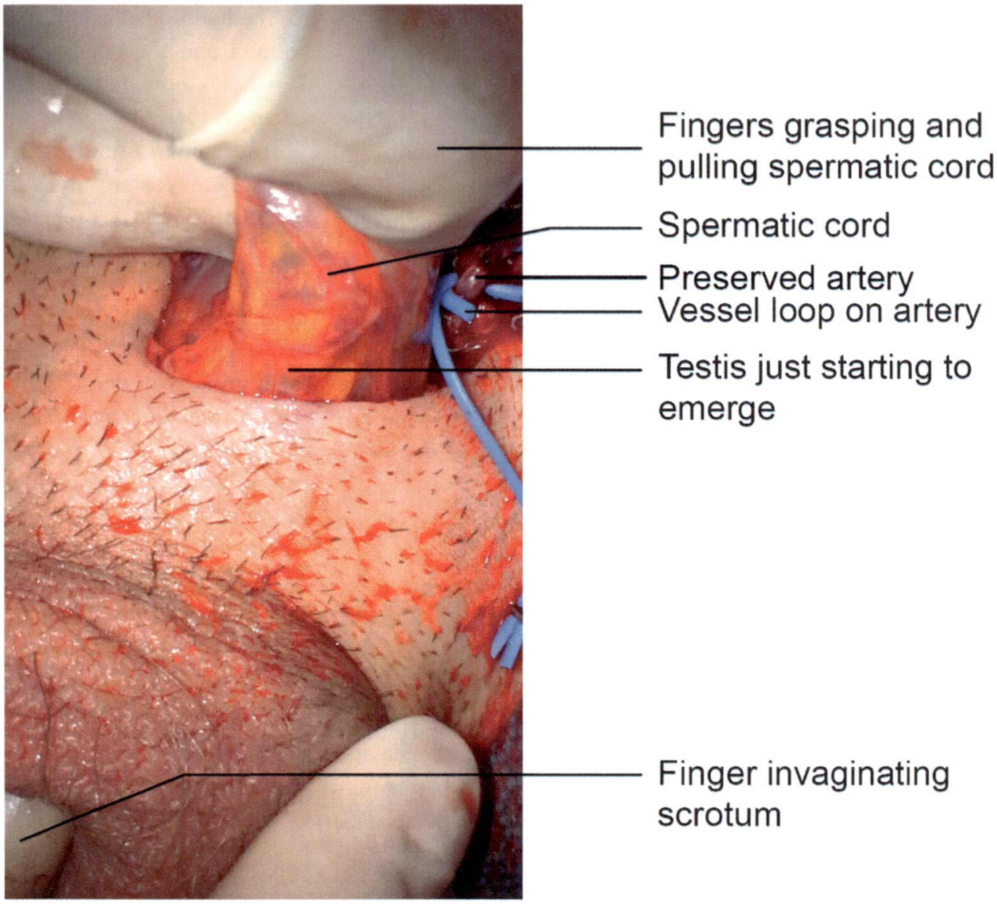

Fig. 3.20 With the left hand, gently pulling on the cord, taking care not to pull on the vessel loops surrounding the arteries, and mostly pushing up on the testes with the middle and index fingers of the right hand, the testis is delivered

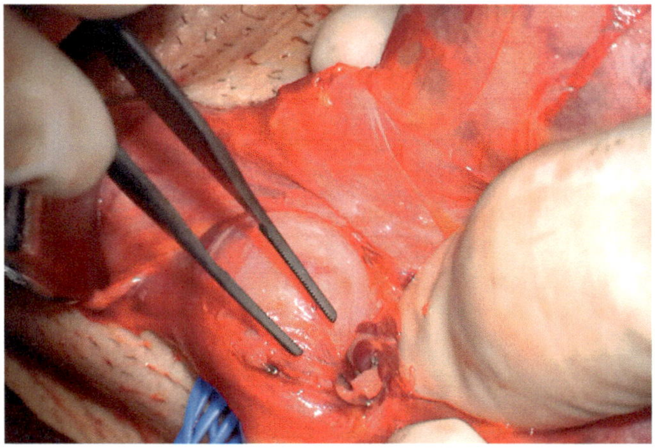

Fig. 3.21 A small Richardson retractor is placed in the lower aspect of the wound, exposing the gubernaculum. This is thinned out with two fingers until the edge of the tunica vaginalis is clearly seen

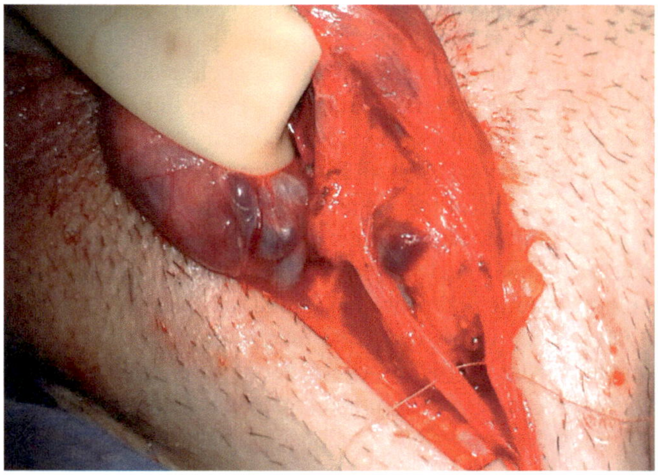

Fig. 3.22 The testis is returned to the scrotum and the cord run again to make sure no additional veins have appeared. The spermatic fascia is reapproximated with interrupted sutures of 5-0 vicryl, pulling up on the suture placed at the apex when the spermatic fascia was initially opened

3.6 Closure

The cord is returned to its bed. Scarpa's fascia is reapproximated with two or three interrupted sutures of 3-0 monofilament absorbable sutures as is Camper's fascia. The subcuticular tissue is reapproximated with two or three interrupted horizontal mattress sutures of 4-0 monofilament absorbable (Fig. 3.23). The wound is infiltrated with Marcaine 2% with epinephrine (Fig. 3.24). The skin is then closed with 5-0 subcuticular monofilament absorbable sutures (Fig. 3.25), reinforced with steri-strips (Fig. 3.26). The thickness of the scar is more related to relieving underlying tension before closing the skin than the perfection of the skin closure. The "Sign of the Fox" is the typical appearance of the wounds following a bilateral varicocelectomy just prior to closure (Fig. 3.27) [6].

Lastly, the testis is pulled down low in the scrotum, so it does not get stuck high up (this has only occurred once in

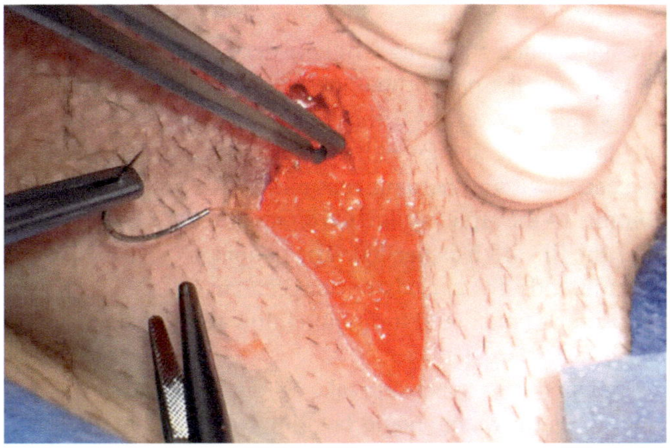

Fig. 3.23 The subcuticular tissue is re-approximated with two or three interrupted horizontal mattress sutures of 4-0 monofilament absorbable

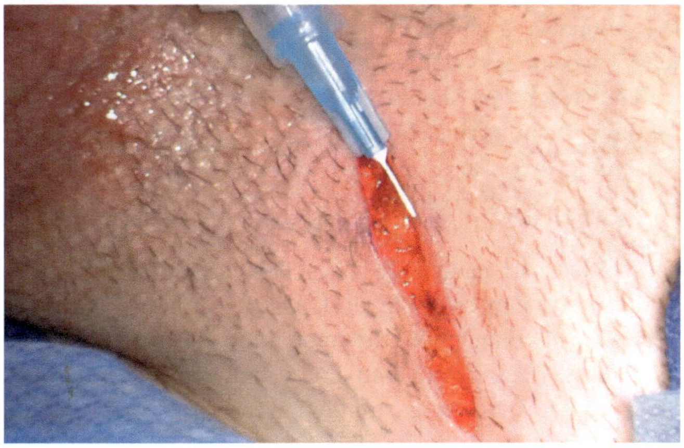

Fig. 3.24 The wound is infiltrated with Marcaine 2% with epinephrine

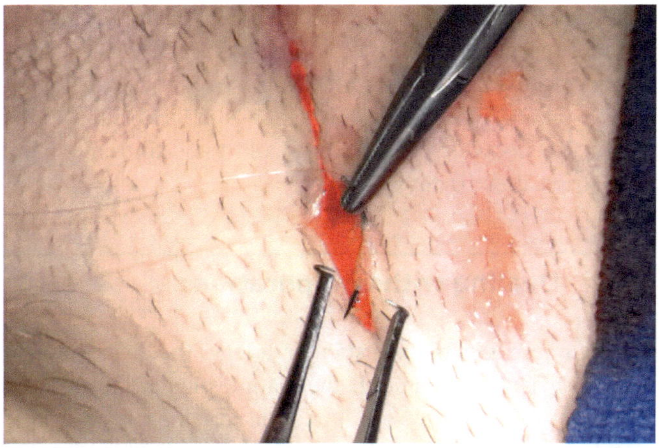

Fig. 3.25 The skin is then closed with 5-0 subcuticular monofilament absorbable sutures

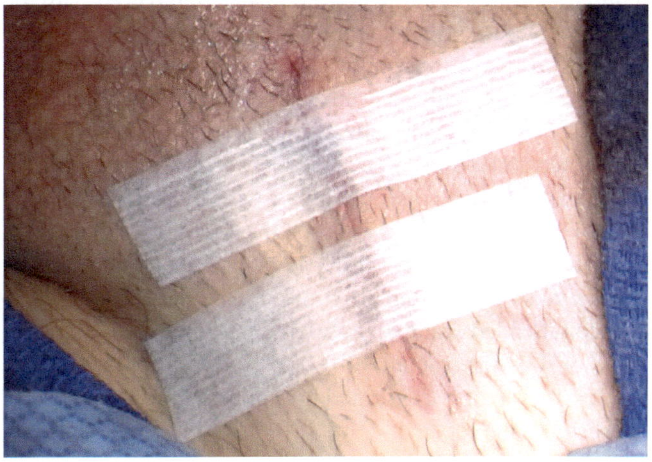

Fig. 3.26 The skin is then reinforced with steri-strips

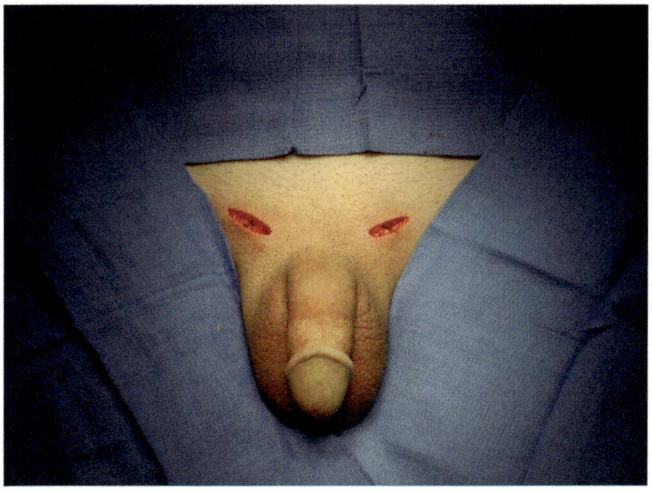

Fig. 3.27 The "Sign of the Fox" is the typical appearance of the wounds following a bilateral varicocelectomy just prior to closure (*From* Goldstein and Li [6]; *with permission*)

5000 cases for me requiring reoperation to bring it down). A scrotal supporter with fluff dressings is placed. A 10 lb. sandbag is placed on the wound for 1 h, followed by ice packs for 20 min on, 10 min off for 48 h. After 48 h have elapsed, the patient can shower. The patient is told they can remove the steri-strips after 10 days.

3.7 Dealing with Complications

If you injure the main testicular artery, the first thing to remember is: don't panic. If the main testicular artery has a hole in it or a partial tear, this is ascertained by pulsatile blood coming from the hole. Most small arterial bleeders are the result of small arterial branches ripped off when cleaning the artery. Very small ones can be sealed with the microbipolar cautery set at low power and/or holding pressure for 5 min on the clock. Large holes or tears are repaired with the same double-armed 10-0 nylon sutures with a tapered needle used for vasovasostomy or vaso-epididymostomy. Compress the artery proximally and have your assistant irrigate continuously to enable visualization of the edges of the hole. Place the sutures inside-out; one or two sutures will usually do the trick. I then cover the repair with Floseal and nearby fat and hold pressure for 5 min on the clock.

If the main testicular artery is completely transected, as evidenced by a pulsating proximal stump, then arterial repair is recommended using a vascular approximating clamp and three to four interrupted 10-0 double-armed nylon sutures. Successful repair is confirmed by a good micro-Doppler signal distal to the repair.

3.8 Postoperative Instructions Given to Our Patients

I tell my patients that it is likely that they will have some discomfort for the first 2–3 weeks after surgery. At the time of discharge from the hospital, I prescribe pain medication and instruct them to be careful while walking or climbing stairs, as dizziness is not unusual while taking pain medication. I also prescribe a course of Celebrex, taken the night prior to surgery and for 6 days thereafter, to help reduce inflammation and decrease dependence on postoperative pain killers.

I explain that swelling and bruising of the penis and scrotum are normal and will take about 3 weeks to mostly resolve. They can expect a hard ridge as if a pencil is buried under the skin where the incision is. This is from the muscles sewn up under the skin and is normal, and this will gradually soften and flatten out over the weeks following surgery. They may feel small bumps or lumps around the upper and lower ends of the incision; these are the surgical knots buried underneath the skin. In time they will shrink, soften, and dissolve. Additionally, the patient may feel a "hardness" or tube-like structures above the testes. This is caused by thrombosis of the varicoceles and should dissolve in approximately 6–12 weeks. Finally, enlarged, hard veins on the penis are normal following the surgery and will resolve in approximately 2–3 weeks.

I warn the patient that a small amount of bright red blood showing through the gauze dressing is to be expected, and to not be alarmed. They can contact the office if they feel the amount is excessive. Bloody gauze can be replaced with clean, but if there is no bleeding, the wound does not need to be covered with the gauze. Additionally, a low-grade fever (up to 100 °F) is common for 2–3 days postoperatively and can be reduced by coughing, deep breathing, and walking. The patient is told that there is no danger that these activities will disrupt the incisions. Taking pain medication for 1 h prior to these activities and placing a pillow over the lower abdomen when coughing will help decrease discomfort.

I instruct the patient to apply ice to the incision for 48 h postoperatively, as this is the preferred treatment for soft tissue injury. Cold therapy will not reduce edema that is already present, but it will help prevent more swelling and ease discomfort on the affected site. Ice compresses can be continued after the first 48 h as needed. The patient should apply them intermittently for periods no longer than 20 min, as longer exposure to cold could limit blood flow to injured tissue and cause secondary damage.

Patients are instructed to take a shower 48 h after the procedure. Warm water should be allowed to run over the incisions, and the wound can be gently washed with soap, being careful not to rub hard or scrub. The steri-strips should be allowed to remain in place and dried gently. The patient should shower daily until their postoperative examination 4 weeks after the procedure, as it is very important to keep the wound area clean. Tub baths should be avoided for at least 1 week postoperatively.

The steri-strips should fall off on their own after about 10 days of showering, but if they have not yet fallen off at that point, they can be gently peeled off with the assistance of a cotton swab soaked in water or an adhesive remover wipe.

Patients who have a job that involves only desk work or light activity may return to work 3–4 days following the surgery, but anything more strenuous and the patient should wait for 1 week postoperatively before returning to work. Heavy work, swimming, strenuous exercise or sports should be avoided for 3 weeks postoperatively. Further, sexual intercourse can be resumed 1 week postoperatively.

I call my surgical patients the day after their procedure to check on them and to review their postoperative instructions. Often, immediately after surgery they do not recall any information I review with them in the recovery room, so I like to follow up with them the next day. I remind them at that time to schedule a 4-week postoperative appointment to check healing and progressive resolution of the varicoceles.

For patients having the varicocele repaired for fertility reasons, I have them do a semen analysis 3 months after surgery, and then every 6 months thereafter until the couple is able to conceive. For patients with pre-operative low testosterone, I have them repeat the total testosterone at the time of their one-month postoperative examination.

Tips [7]

- If you are not sure if a vessel is a vein or a lymphatic, squeeze on the scrotal pampiniform plexus. If it is a vein, it will fill with blood. Recheck at the very end of the ligation and if the squeeze test is still uncertain, ligate it rather than risk recurrence. There are many lymphatics and ligating one will not cause a hydrocele.
- Always look for clean edges of arteries and veins.
- When tying veins, never pull up!! Bring the knot down to the vessel.

References

1. Beck E, Schlegel P, Goldstein M. Intraoperative varicocele anatomy: a macroscopic and microscopic study. J Urol. 1992;148(4):1190–4.
2. Schiff J, et al. Managing varicoceles in children: results with microsurgical varicocelectomy. BJU Int. 2005;95(3):399–402.
3. Goldstein M, et al. Microsurgical inguinal varicocelectomy with delivery of the testis: an artery and lymphatic sparing technique. J Urol. 1992;148(6):1808–11.
4. Amelar R, Dubin L, Walsh P. Male infertility. London: Saunders; 1977.
5. Dabaja A, Goldstein M. Microsurgical hydrocelectomy: rationale and technique. Urol Pract. 2014;1(4):189–93.
6. Goldstein M, Li P. Sign of the fox. Urology. 2008;73:499.
7. Partin AW, Wein AJ, Kavoussi LR, Peters CA, Dmochowski, RR. Campbell Walsh Wein Urology, EBook. Elsevier Health Sciences; 2020.

4 Microsurgical Hydrocelectomy

The most satisfying hydrocelectomy I ever performed was on a man that developed a HUGE hydrocele after an unsuccessful previous varicocelectomy. The whole scrotum was filled with fluid the size of a softball. After repairing it, the pain and discomfort disappeared. More importantly, after being virtually azoospermic, he got good sperm back and his wife conceived naturally. The first sperm he got back was enough to use IVF, and they had their first baby that way. He had several more children after that, all conceived naturally.

4.1 Introduction

A hydrocele is a collection of serous fluid within the tunica vaginalis (Fig. 4.1) and can present as non-communicating, communicating, or hydrocele of the spermatic cord (Fig. 4.2). This can have an insulating effect and negatively impact testicular function [1]. Microsurgical hydrocelectomy minimizes the risk of injury to the epididymis, vas deferens, and/or testicular blood supply, as well as the risk of infection or hematoma [2].

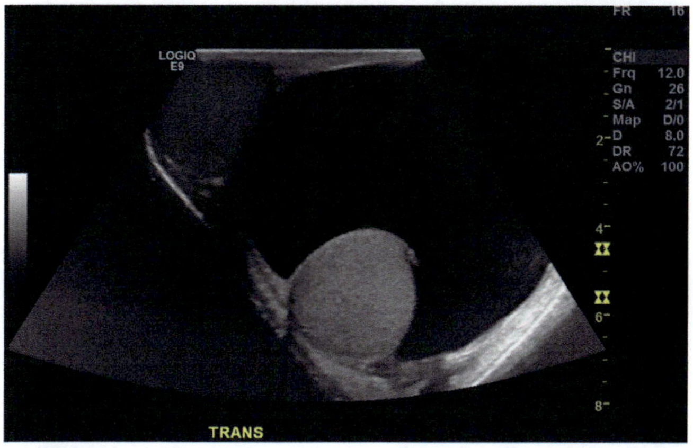

Fig. 4.1 A hydrocele is a collection of serous fluid within the tunica vaginalis

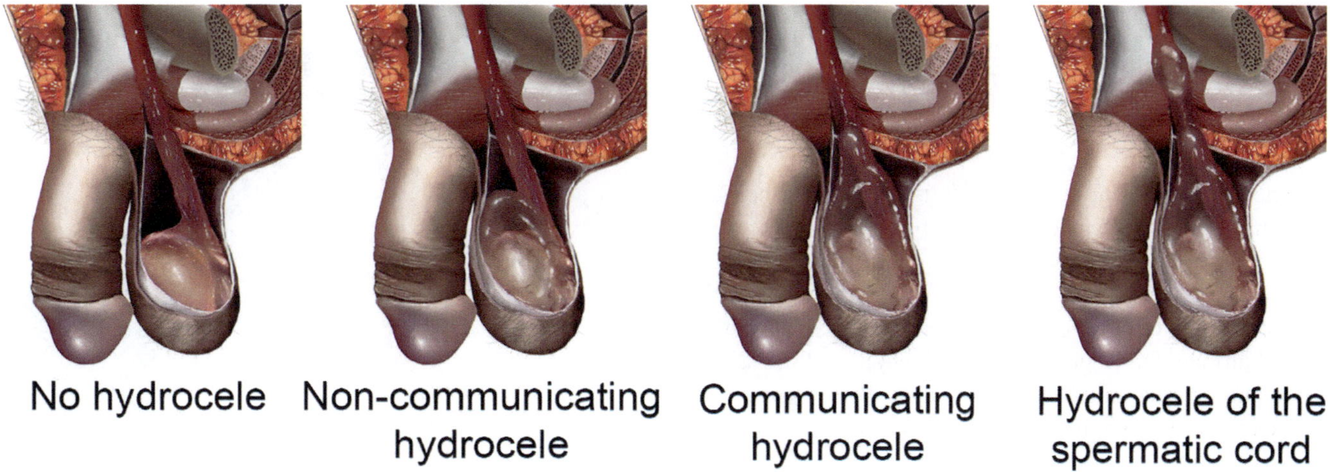

Fig. 4.2 A hydrocele can present as non-communicating, communicating, or hydrocele of the spermatic cord

M. Goldstein, *Atlas of Male Infertility Microsurgery*, https://doi.org/10.1007/978-3-031-31601-2_4

4.2 Procedure

Hydrocelectomy begins with a scrotal incision. Mark the median raphe as a reference point, then use a transverse scrotal skinfold incision (Fig. 4.3). Using a Bovie electrocautery, divide the dartos muscle and control bleeders (Fig. 4.4). Both sharp and blunt dissection are used to dissect the hydrocele out of the scrotum and the inguinal canal, until it can be cleanly delivered (Fig. 4.5). The dissection is continued up toward the inguinal canal. Large veins are doubly clamped, tied, and ligated (Fig. 4.6). Using a retractor to expose the spermatic cord and identify the vas deferens (Fig. 4.7a, b), the spermatic cord is dissected, identifying the internal spermatic fascia and its enclosed vessels, and the vas. The internal spermatic fascia with its vessels is isolated with a Penrose drain, and the vas is dissected free from the adherent fascia, and isolated with a small Penrose drain (Fig. 4.8). Once the entire hydrocele is delivered, pick an avascular spot and poke (Fig. 4.9). The hydrocele sac is opened with the Bovie anteriorly away from the testes and epididymis. The sac is everted (Fig. 4.10), and the testis is delivered (Fig. 4.11). The vas and epididymis can often be within the sac walls. The sac is resected leaving a 1–2 cm margin around the epididymis. The operating microscope is used to visualize the vas and epididymis. The sac is completely resected, and the circumference is cauterized. Finally, the edges of the remaining sac is over-sewn with continuous 4-0 chromic catgut sutures. The over-sewn sac is everted, and a bottleneck is performed with continuous 2-0 PDS (Fig. 4.12a–c). This will prevent anterior re-approximation of the tunica vaginalis causing a

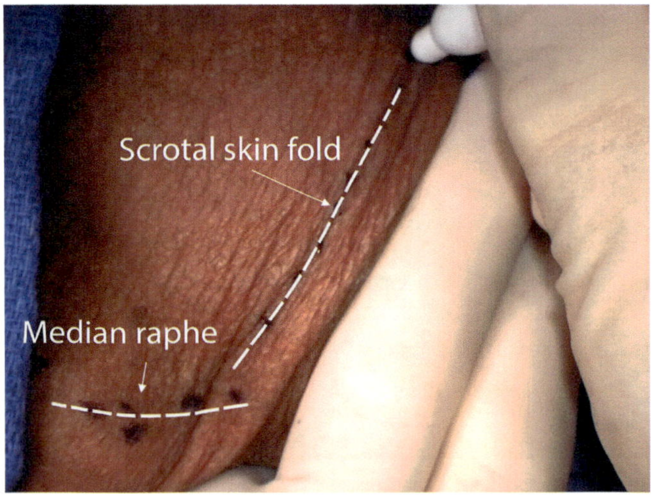

Fig. 4.3 Mark the median raphe as a reference point, then use a transverse scrotal skinfold incision

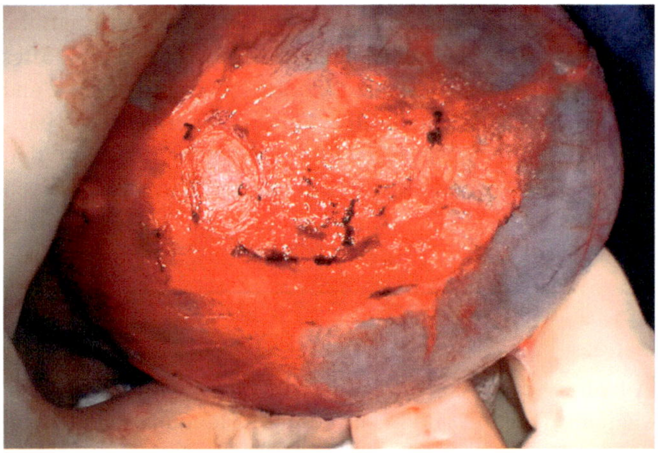

Fig. 4.5 Both sharp and blunt dissection are used to dissect the hydrocele out of the scrotum and the inguinal canal, until it can be cleanly delivered

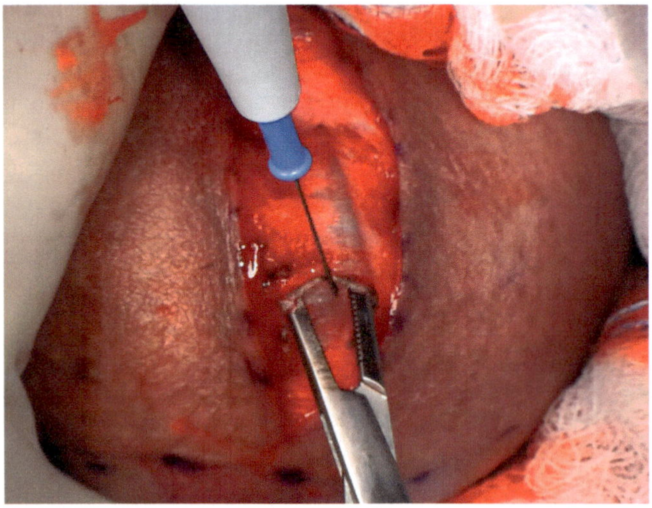

Fig. 4.4 Using a Bovie electrocautery, divide the dartos muscle and control bleeders

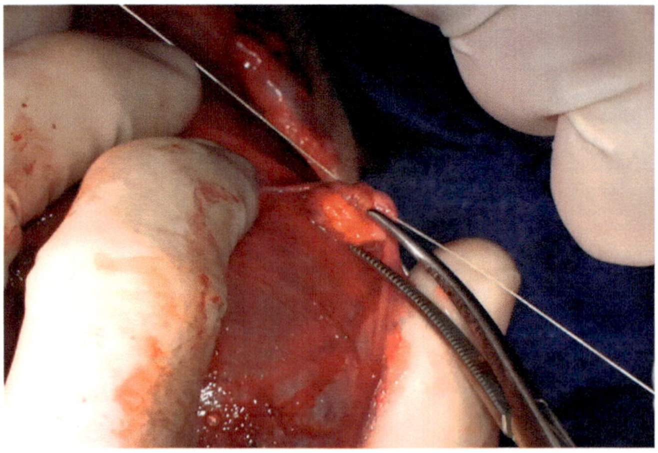

Fig. 4.6 The dissection is continued up toward the inguinal canal. Large veins are doubly clamped, tied, and ligated

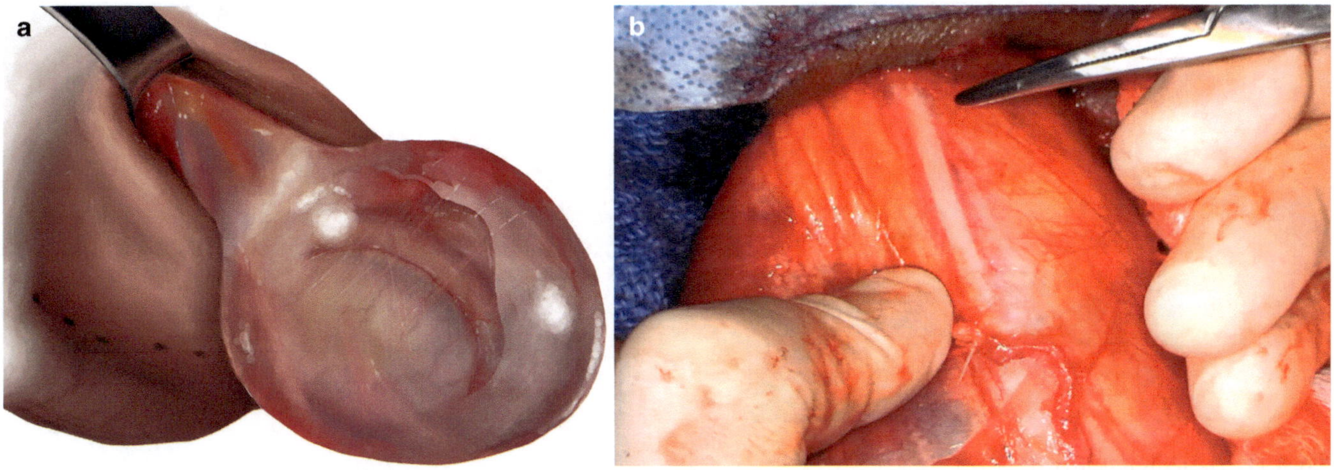

Fig. 4.7 (**a, b**) Using a retractor to expose the spermatic cord and identify the vas deferens, the spermatic cord is dissected, identifying the pampiniform plexus and vas

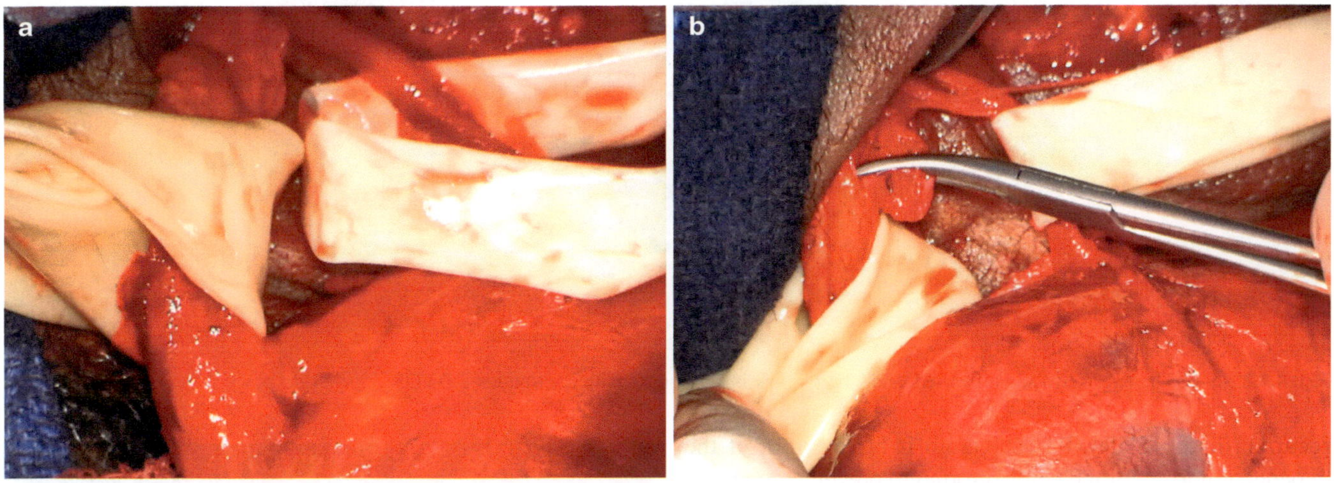

Fig. 4.8 (**a, b**) The pampiniform plexus is isolated with a Penrose drain, and the vas is dissected free from adherent fascia, and isolated with a small Penrose drain

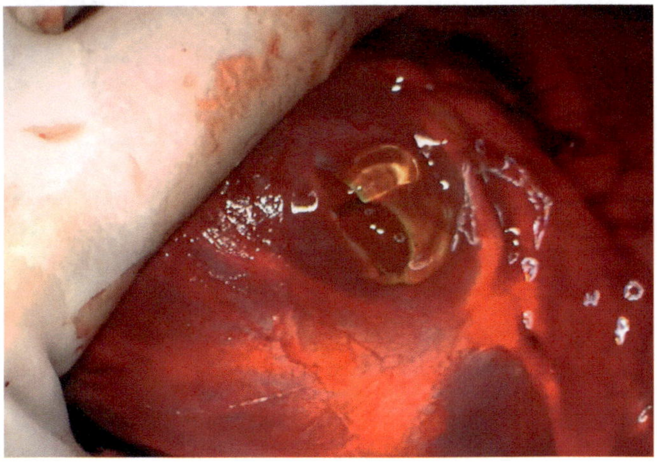

Fig. 4.9 Once the entire hydrocele is exposed, pick an avascular spot and poke. The hydrocele sac is open anteriorly away from the testes and epididymis

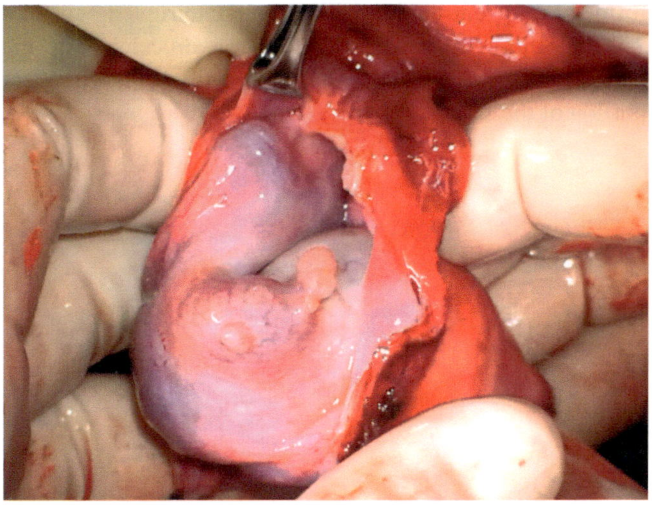

Fig. 4.10 The sac is everted

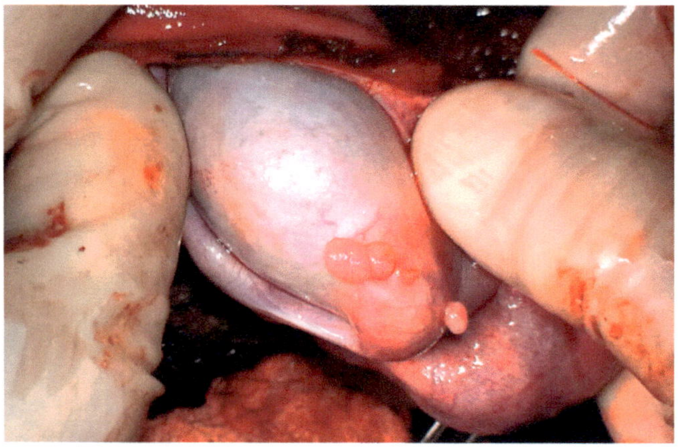

Fig. 4.11 The testis is delivered

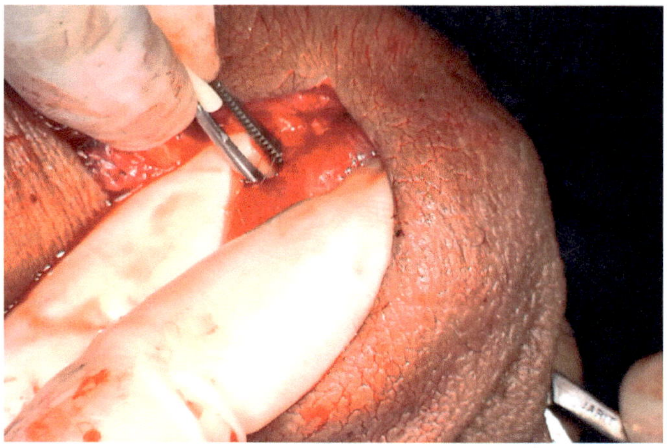

Fig. 4.13 A Penrose drain is brought out of the dependent portion of the hemi-scrotum to prevent hematoma

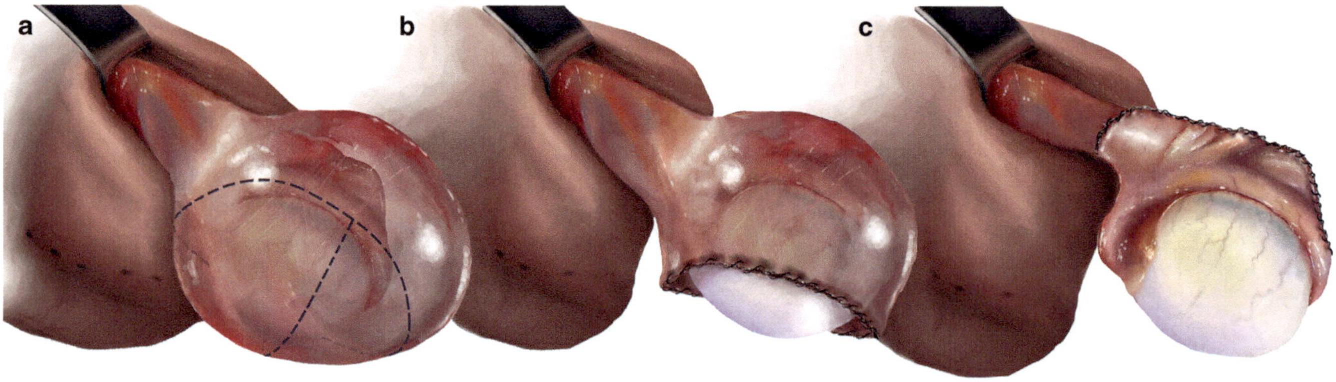

Fig. 4.12 (**a–c**) The over-sewn sac is everted, and a bottleneck is performed with continuous 2-0 PDS

recurrent hydrocele. A Penrose drain is brought out of the dependent portion of the hemi-scrotum to prevent hematoma (Fig. 4.13) and is fixed in place with 2-0 Silk and a safety pin (Fig. 4.14), after which the testis is returned to the scrotum. When the hydrocele is very large, fixation of the testis is performed to prevent torsion with a three interrupted suture of 2-0 PDS through the edges of the cut hydrocele sac to the dartos muscle, the testis is then replaced in the dependent portion of the scrotum.

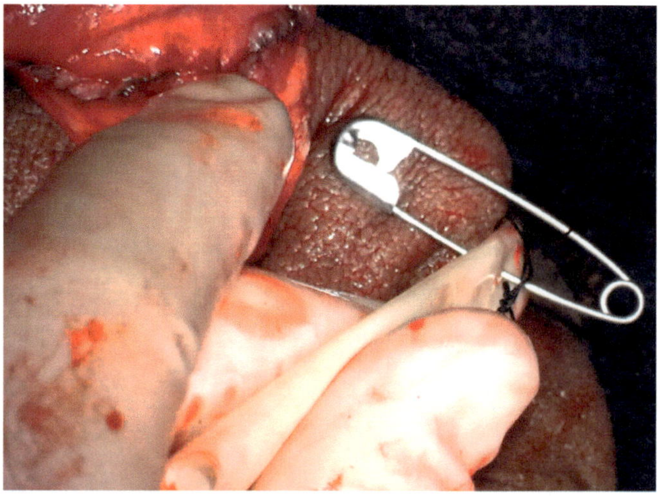

Fig. 4.14 A Penrose drain is fixed in place with 2-0 Silk and a safety pin

4.3 Closure

The dartos is reapproximated with a 4-0 biosyn. The wound is infiltrated with 0.25% Marcaine. The skin is closed with a subcuticular suture, a 5-0 Monocryl. Done correctly, the incision should be hidden between the scrotal skin folds. Bacitracin ointment is applied to the wound and sterile dressings are held in place with a scrotal supporter. The patient is able to remove their drains at home 24–48 h following the surgery.

Tips

I have never regretted putting in a drain; I have only ever regretted not leaving a drain.

Transillumination of a thick-walled hydrocele sac will help identify the vas and/or epididymis within the wall of the sac.

4.4 Postoperative Instructions

Other than providing patients with instructions for drain removal, the postoperative instructions provided to patients for hydrocelectomy are the same as in varicocelectomy.

References

1. Dabaja A, Goldstein M. Microsurgical hydrocelectomy: rationale and technique. Urol Pract. 2014;1(4):189–93.
2. Hopps CV, Goldstein M. Microsurgical reconstruction of iatrogenic injuries to the epididymis from hydrocelectomy. J Urol. 2006;176:2077–80.

Microsurgical Spermatocelectomy

5

5.1 Introduction

A spermatocele is a sperm-containing cystic structure at the superior aspect of the epididymis (Fig. 5.1). It is essentially an aneurysm arising from a 150 μ diameter efferent duct. It may be caused or exacerbated by distal obstruction, such as vasectomy. Physical examination reveals a soft transilluminable well-defined cystic mass at the head of the epididymis. A scrotal ultrasound will reveal a hypoechoic simple cyst at the epididymal head (Fig. 5.2). The largest spermatocele I ever encountered was in a 58-year-old male and physical examination revealed a tense, transilluminable 15 cm × 8 cm × 8 cm scrotal mass, with the testis at the inferior aspect of it. It was recognizable as a spermatocele rather than a hydrocele, as the testis would instead be in the middle of the sac.

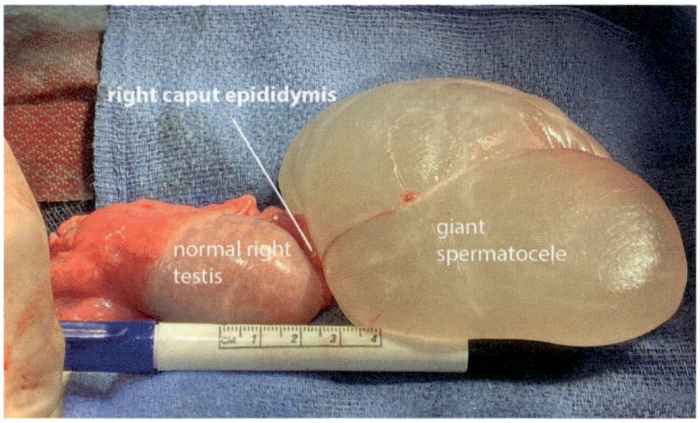

Fig. 5.1 A spermatocele is a sperm-containing cystic structure at the superior aspect of the epididymis

Spermatoceles are found in approximately 30% of asymptomatic men who undergo scrotal ultrasound for other reasons. Pain or discomfort due to large size is a primary indication for intervention. Magnification with an operating microscope reduces the risk of epididymal injury and other complications associated with spermatocelectomy [1]. The microscope facilitates dissection of the spermatocele and allows for clear identification of the spermatocele neck for ligation.

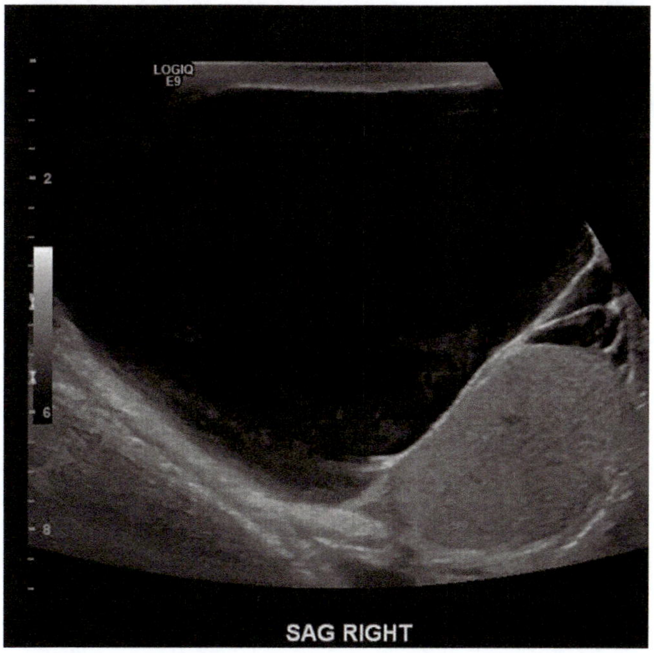

Fig. 5.2 A scrotal ultrasound will reveal a hypoechoic simple cyst at the epididymal head

M. Goldstein, *Atlas of Male Infertility Microsurgery*, https://doi.org/10.1007/978-3-031-31601-2_5

5.2 Procedure Description

The spermatocele is approached through a transverse scrotal incision within the scrotal skin folds, similarly to the initial incision for hydrocelectomy (*see* Fig. 4.3). The size of the incision depends on the size of the spermatocele. The tunica vaginalis is opened with electrocautery. The testis and spermatocele is delivered into the operative field (Fig. 5.3). The spermatocele is carefully dissected away from the surrounding epididymis using sharp micro-scissor dissection, along with bipolar cautery. Gentle blunt dissection may also be used. Irrigation with lactated ringer's solution and bipolar electrocautery maintain hemostasis; the other side of the spermatocele is dissected in a similar fashion. Although many scrotal procedures involve the risk of epididymal injury, the risk is elevated during spermatocelectomy because of its origin from, and close proximity to, the epididymal tubules. The excised spermatocele is aspirated with a 30-gauge needle attached to a tuberculin syringe. A sample of spermatocele fluid is glass slide with a cover slip and examined under 400 power magnification using a separate bench microscope. The presence of many sperm with variable motility confirms the diagnosis of spermatocele. The isolated efferent duct is ligated with 5-0 Vicryl. The tunica of the epididymis is re-approximated to the tunica albuginea with interrupted 5-0 Vicryl sutures. The testis and epididymis are returned to the tunica vaginalis which is closed with a continuous 5-0 Vicryl suture. The testis is returned to the scrotum and the dartos and skin are closed in separate layers. For large or complex spermatoceles, a Penrose drain is brought out of the dependent portion of the hemi-scrotum (*see* Fig. 4.13) and fixed in place with a 2-0 silk stitch and safety pin (*see* Fig. 4.14). The drain is removed in 24–48 h.

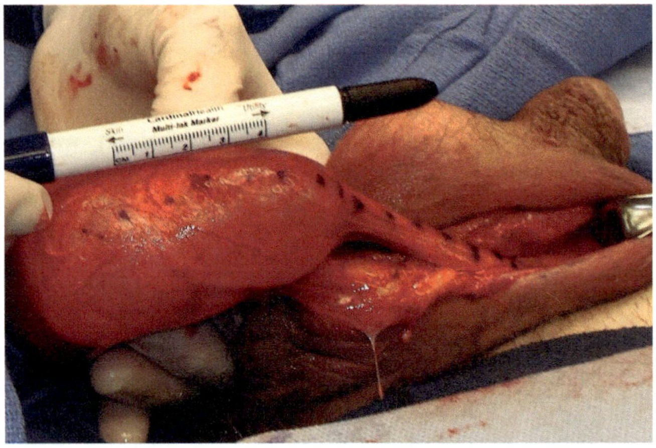

Fig. 5.3 The tunica vaginalis is opened with electrocautery. The testis and spermatocele are delivered into the operative field

Tips

1. Use a blunt curved micro-scissor or Wescott scissor and a micro-needle holder to do the dissection.
2. Use the micro-bipolar to cauterize all bleeders before cutting.
3. Try not to enter the spermatocele until it is completely dissected out. If a small hole is made during the dissection, cauterize it or clamp and tie it.

5.3 Postoperative Instructions

The postoperative instructions for patients undergoing spermatocelectomy are the same as those going through hydrocelectomy or varicocelectomy.

Reference

1. Kaufmann E, et al. Microsurgical spermatocelectomy: technique and outcomes of a novel surgical approach. J Urol. 2011;185:238–42.

6 No-Scalpel Vasectomy

6.1 Introduction

Vasectomy is a widely utilized long-term contraceptive method for men. Vasectomy failure may occur secondary to recanalization and is a major cause of malpractice suits and unwanted pregnancy. The no-scalpel vasectomy is a minimally invasive procedure in which failure rates are dependent on occlusion methods. The puncture-first no-scalpel vasectomy with multi-occlusion techniques minimizes failure and complications. I was the first American surgeon to be trained in and perform the Chinese method of No-Scalpel Vasectomy (NSV), which I introduced to American surgeons in the 1980s [1]. I have since further refined the technique to include no-needle anesthesia using a jet injector [2].

6.2 The Vasectomy Consultation

In New York State, patients are required to have a consultation at least 30 days prior to having a sterilization procedure. At the time of consultation, I review with the patient their options for anesthesia, local and managed anesthesia care. The vast majority of my patients have this procedure done under local anesthesia, some with 10 mg of oral diazepam 1 h prior to the procedure for anxiety. Occasionally, patients will have particularly difficult anatomy: difficult to palpate vasa, excessive fat surrounding the pubis, or scar tissue from previous scrotal procedures which would make performing this procedure under local anesthesia difficult. For these patients, I generally recommend managed anesthesia care (MAC), similar to that used for colonoscopy. The postoperative care is the same, but having the patient under sedation relaxes the scrotum, allowing easier access to the vasa.

6.3 Procedure Description

The patient is prepped by shaving the scrotum and using a rubber band around the penis to secure it up and away from the scrotum. Betadine is used to prep the site and then wiped away with alcohol after draping. We do not routinely give patient antibiotics. The first step is to identify the median raphe (Fig. 6.1) and avoid any scrotal blood vessels which are superficial and may bleed. The ideal entry site is found in the median raphe at the midway point from the top of the testis to the base of the penis (Fig. 6.2). The three-finger technique is used to isolate the vas (Fig. 6.3). The goal of the isolation is to ensure that the vas is placed under the small mark that we made in the median raphe (Fig. 6.4). This will ensure that only one puncture site is used for both sides. The middle finger of the left hand is placed beneath the scrotum

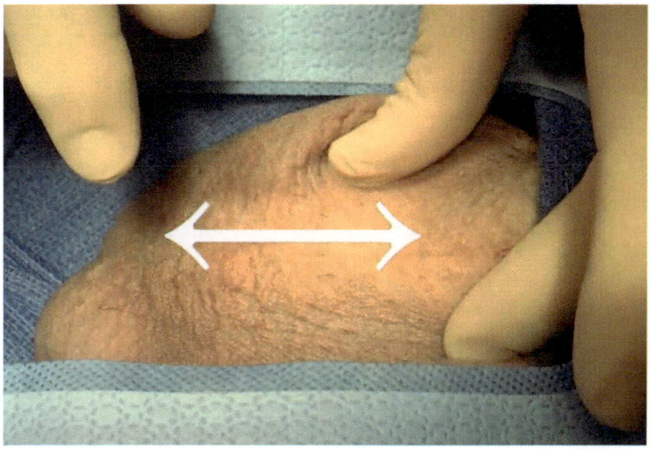

Fig. 6.1 Identify the median raphe and avoid any scrotal blood vessels which are superficial and may bleed

M. Goldstein, *Atlas of Male Infertility Microsurgery*, https://doi.org/10.1007/978-3-031-31601-2_6

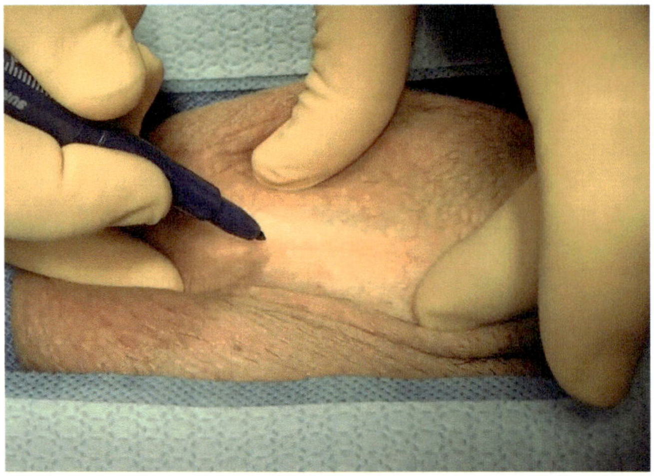

Fig. 6.2 The ideal entry site is found in the median raphe at the midway point from the top of the testis to the base of the penis

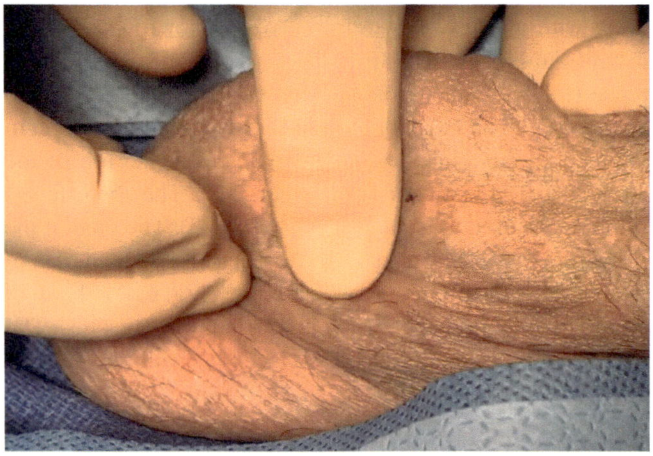

Fig. 6.3 The three-finger technique is used to isolate the vas

and the spermatic cord structures are drawn from the midline laterally until the vas deferens is trapped between the middle finger, the thumb, and the index finger. The location of the thumb is just below the optimal puncture site. The middle finger elevates and isolates the vas while the index finger stabilizes the vas. The nerve block can be performed in various ways. We use a jet injector device that injects a high-pressure mist of lidocaine without epinephrine solution under the skin (Item# 401UR, MadaMedical, Carlstaft, NJ) (Fig. 6.5). For those that are inexperienced in using this device, a finger protector should be used to avoid inadvertently anesthetizing the finger. The same jet injector is used to deliver anesthesia to the left side after isolating the vas under the same mark previously made. Another way to deliver the nerve block is using a conventional needle and a controller syringe. A 30-gauge 1½ in needle is inserted at a 45° angle where first a wheel is raised over the intended puncture site, on top of the vas deferens (Fig. 6.6). The needle is then advanced along the vas deferens within the vasal sheath toward the external ring delivering 300–500 μL of local anesthetic. Three finger fixation is again used to isolate the vas. The scrotal skin and vas wall are punctured using one blade of the sharp curved hemostat introduced at a 45° angle down toward the lumen of the vas (Fig. 6.7). The tips of the curved hemostat are then closed and reintroduced into the puncture hole. The skin and vasal sheath are spread, revealing the bare vas and even its lumen (Fig. 6.8). The exposed vas is regrasped with the ring clamp to keep it from falling back into the scrotum (Fig. 6.9). This technique is technically less challenging than using the ring forceps to grasp both the scrotal skin and the vas as in the original no-scalpel vasectomy technique. Once the vas is lifted to the skin with the ring clamp, a sharp curved hemostat with serration filed off (the dissection clamp) is used to skewer the vas (Fig. 6.10). The blade is inserted into the vasal wall and then rotated 180° (Fig. 6.11). The vas is then

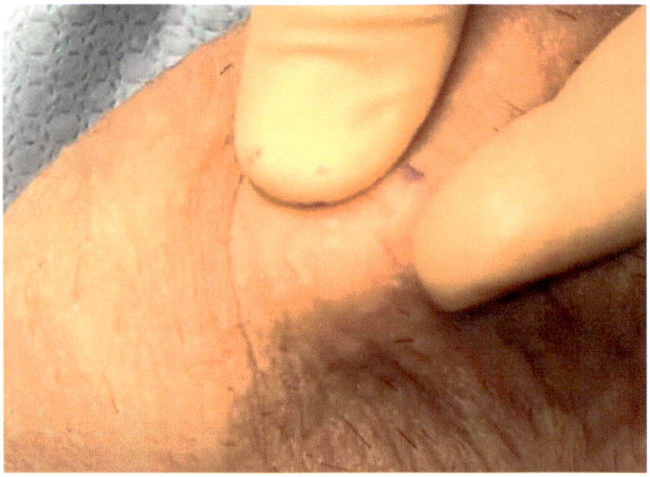

Fig. 6.4 The goal of the isolation is to ensure that the vas is placed under the small mark that we made in the median raphe

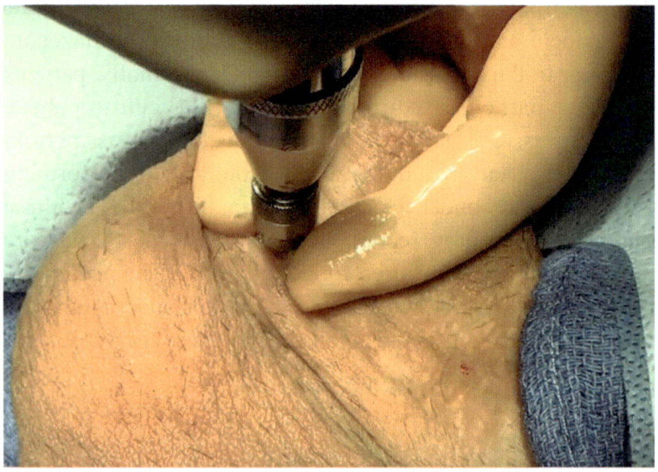

Fig. 6.5 A jet injector device injects a high-pressure mist of lidocaine without epinephrine solution under the skin

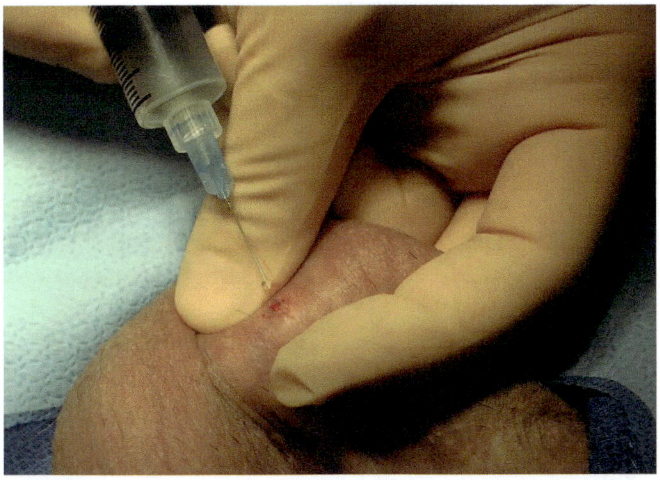

Fig. 6.6 A 30-gauge 1½ in. needle is inserted at a 45° angle where first a wheel is raised over the intended puncture site, on top of the vas deferens

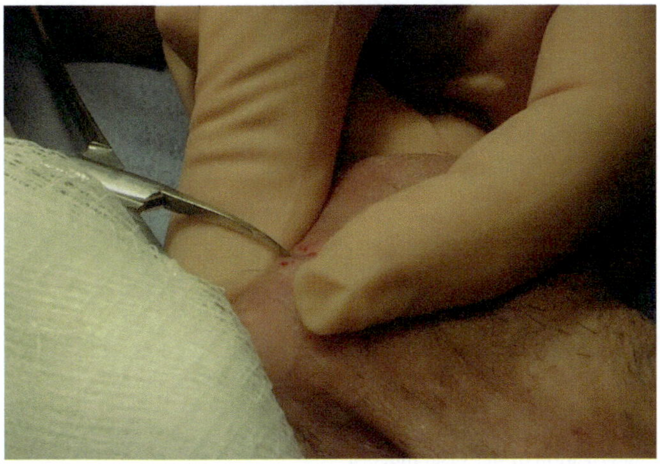

Fig. 6.7 The scrotal skin and vas wall are punctured using one blade of the sharp curved hemostat introduced at a 45° angle down toward the lumen of the vas

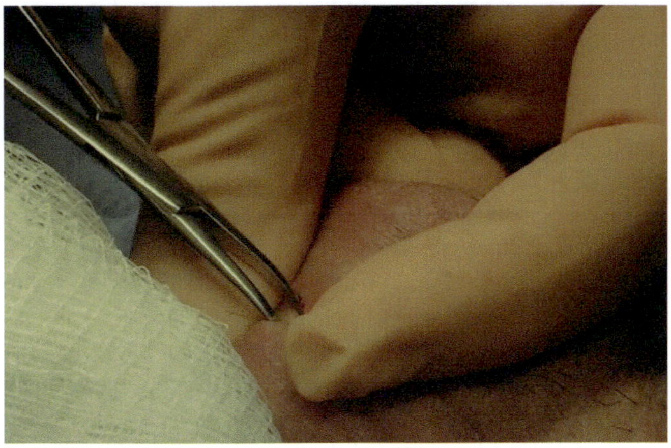

Fig. 6.8 The tips of the curved hemostat are then closed and reintroduced into the puncture hole. The skin and vasal sheath are spread, revealing the bare vas and its lumen

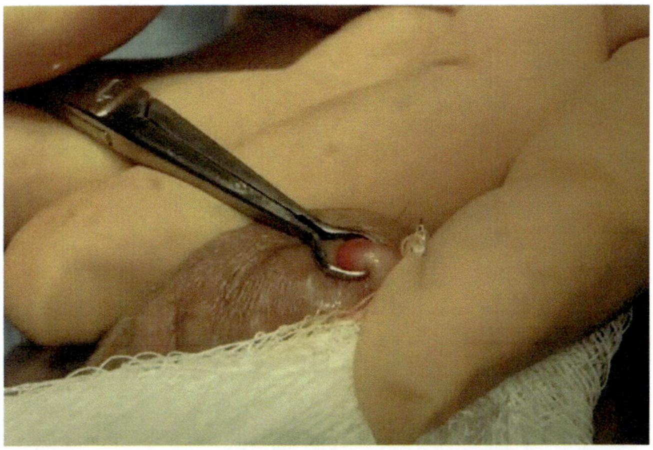

Fig. 6.9 The exposed vas is regrasped with the ring clamp to keep it from falling back into the scrotum

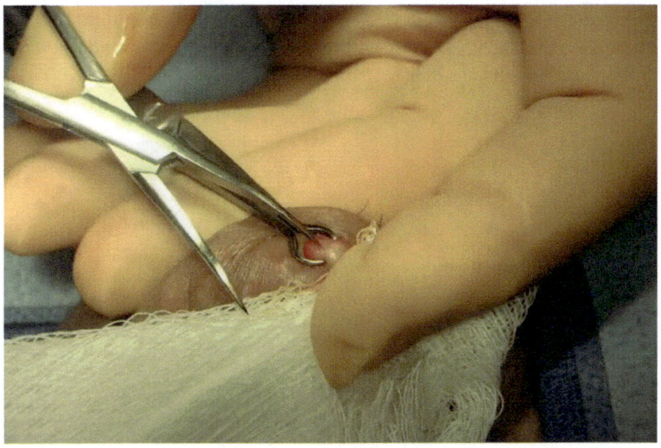

Fig. 6.10 Once the vas is lifted to the skin with the ring clamp, a sharp curved hemostat with serration filed off (the dissection clamp) is used to skewer the vas

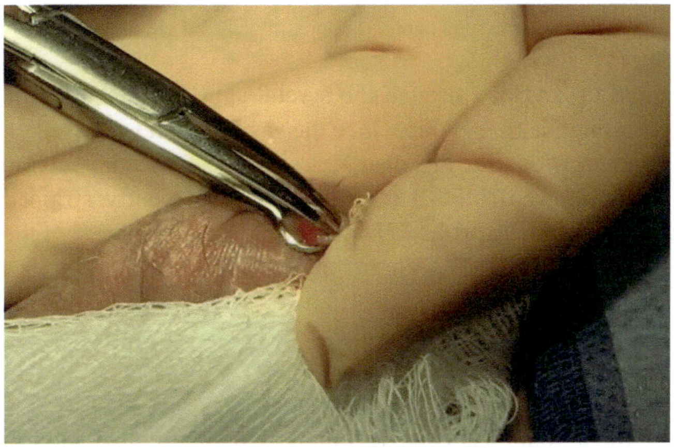

Fig. 6.11 The blade is inserted into the vasal wall and then rotated 180°

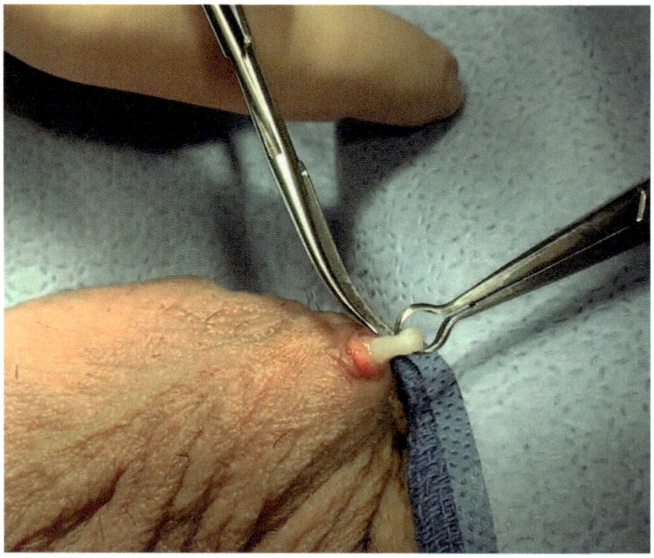

Fig. 6.12 Once the vas is free, it is then again secured with the ring clamp and the sheath and, using the dissecting clamp, spreading vertically, vasal vessels are gently stripped from the vas

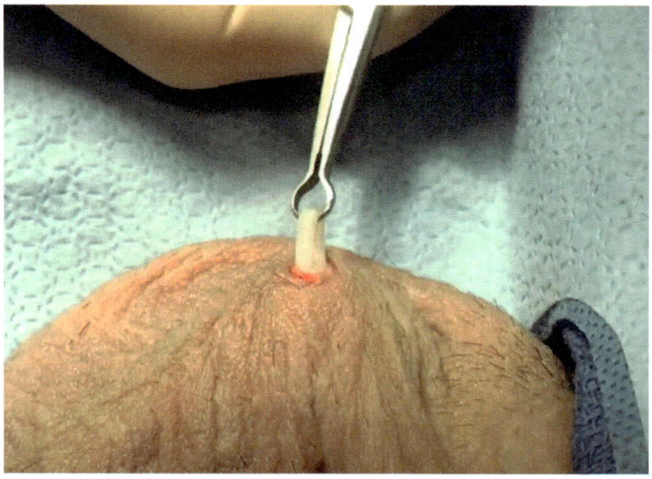

Fig. 6.13 A bare segment of vas approximately 1.5 cm in length

lifted up and out through the scrotal skin at the same time releasing the ring clamp. Once the vas is free, it is then again secured with the ring clamp. Using the dissecting clamp spreading vertically, the vasal vessels are gently stripped from the vas (Fig. 6.12). This will yield a bare segment of the vas approximately 1.5 cm in length (Fig. 6.13).

6.4 Occlusion Techniques

I utilize four occlusion techniques to minimalize failure; intralumenal cautery is used first. A 1 cm cautery tip is used to hemi-transect the vas while holding it with the ring clamp

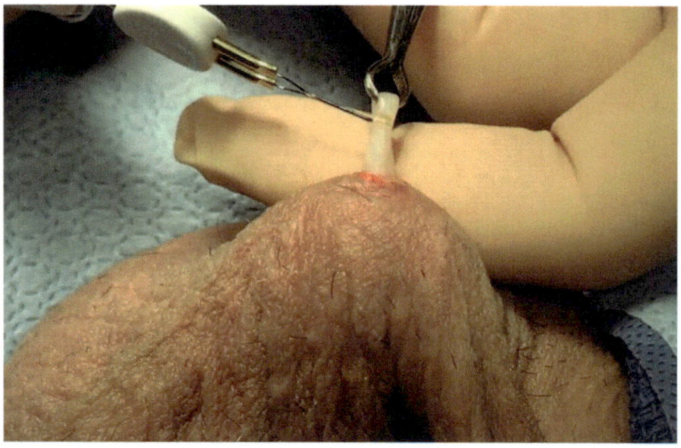

Fig. 6.14 A 1 cm cautery tip is used to hemi-transect the vas while holding it with the ring clamp

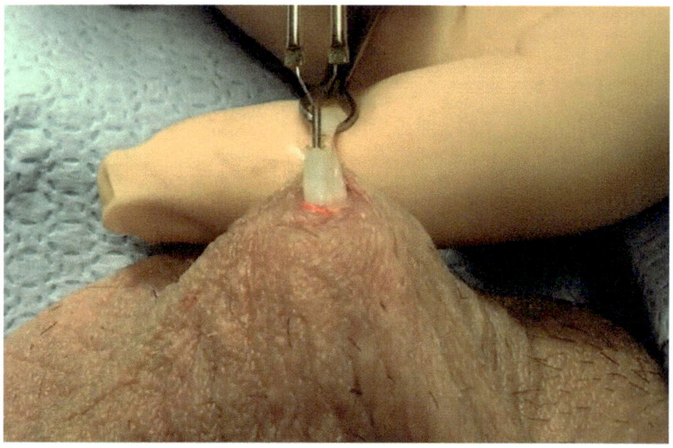

Fig. 6.15 The thermal tip is them inserted into the testicular side of the vas for 10 s while rotating the wires until smoke is seen to ensure 360° cauterization of the vasal mucosa

(Fig. 6.14). The thermal tip is them inserted into the testicular side of the vas for 10 s while rotating the wires until smoke is seen to ensure 360° cauterization of the vasal mucosa (Fig. 6.15). A hemo-clip is then placed lightly on the testicular end to prevent sperm leakage until the cautery eventually causes a permanent seal (Fig. 6.16). The same procedure is performed on the abdominal end of the vas. A small straight clamp is used to grab the middle segment of vas which is then fully transected (Fig. 6.17). Betadine is applied after each step. The vasal sheath is brought over the end of the abdominal vas and secured with a clip (Fig. 6.18); this provides fascial interposition. We then pull on the vas to see the testis move and to ensure that the correct vas was treated. We pull on the testis to pull the vas back into the scrotum, holding onto the testicular end, to see if there is any bleeding. Because the puncture wound is so small it may tamponade any bleeding while the vas is pulled up. Once

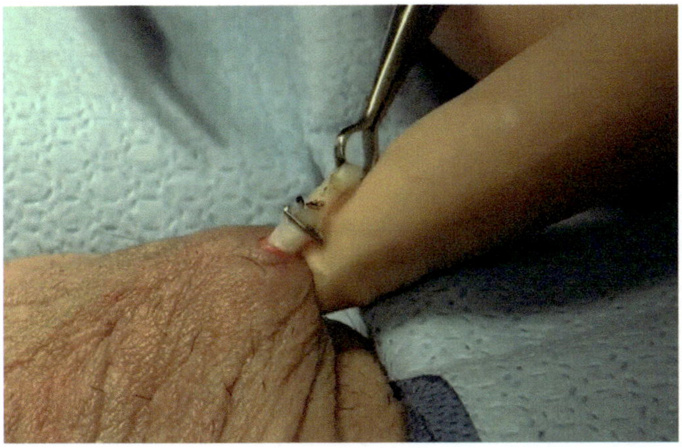

Fig. 6.16 A hemo-clip is then placed lightly on the testicular end to prevent sperm leakage until the cautery eventually causes a permanent seal

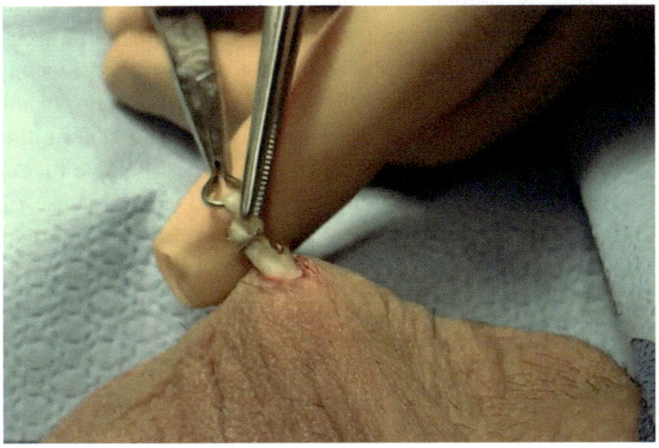

Fig. 6.17 The same procedure is performed on the abdominal end of the vas. A small straight clamp is used to grab the middle segment of vas which is then fully transected

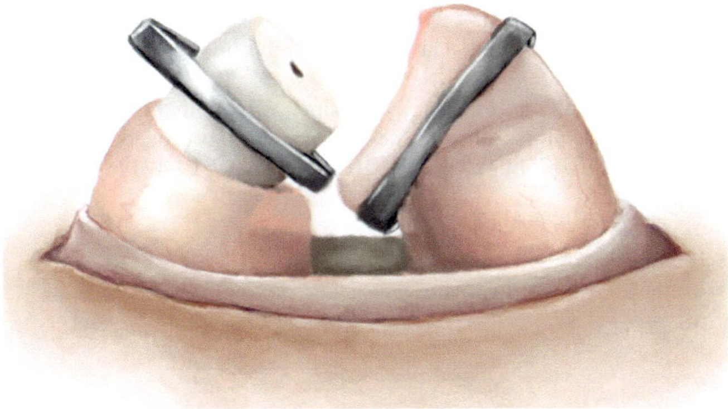

Fig. 6.18 Betadine is applied after each step. The vasal sheath is brought over the end of the abdominal vas and secured with a clip. (*From* Chiles and Goldstein [6]; *with permission*)

bleeding is ruled out, the vas is fully transected between the two clips. After the first vas is placed back into the scrotum, an identical procedure is performed on the contralateral vas through the same puncture hole. Following the bilateral vasectomy, the scrotum is cleaned. Pressure is held on the wound for a minute. Sutures are almost never needed. The puncture hole contracts and is covered with antibiotic ointment and a scrotal support, which holds fluff dressing in place.

Tips

The battery-driven cautery is useful for touching up skin and dartos bleeders at the end of the procedure (BEAVER-VISITEC 1, Manufacturer # 8441500, Cautery, Accu-Temp Hi Temp, ½" shaft).

6.5 Simultaneous Vasectomy and Varicocelectomy

Although infrequently indicated, simultaneous varicocelectomy at the time of vasectomy may be recommended for men presenting for vasectomy with incidentally detected palpable large varicoceles associated with ipsilateral testicular pain or atrophy and for men with symptoms of androgen deficiency or persistent low or low-normal testosterone levels.

When varicocelectomy is properly performed, the deferential veins become the only avenue for testicular venous return. Simultaneous vasectomy-varicocelectomy should therefore be performed microsurgically to identify and ligate both spermatic veins and vasa deferentia. This preserves deferential veins, minimizing the risk of testicular congestion from inadequate venous drainage [3].

6.6 Post-vasectomy Instructions for Patients

The postoperative instructions for vasectomy whether under local anesthesia or MAC are the same. Patients are instructed to apply an ice pack intermittently to the scrotum for 24–48 h following the procedure to decrease discomfort and swelling. I warn the patient that some scrotal swelling and bruising is common and will resolve in a few days. I let them know that a dull ache in the testicles and groin is typical and prescribe the patient ketorolac postoperatively for management of pain, although I tell them that if they prefer to use something over the counter, extra-strength acetaminophen is acceptable. The best way to manage postoperative pain, though, is use of the scrotal supporter. I tell patients to wear the scrotal supporter at all times, even when sleeping, for 48 h after the procedure. They can remove it to shower, but showering should wait for 24 h after the procedure. After the 48 h, though, use of the scrotal supporter can address testicular discomfort, so I recommend patients wear it as needed. I tell patients to refrain from heavy work, exercise, sports, and any sexual activity for one week postoperatively.

A sperm granuloma may form at the vasectomy site over time as a result of the body's immune response to sperm leaking from the cut end of the vas, and this is typically treated with anti-inflammatories.

Of utmost importance, though, is patients need to be counseled that they will not be sterile immediately following the procedure. Semen analysis must be performed either 6 weeks following the procedure, or after 15 ejaculations, whichever comes first. Until semen analysis confirms azoospermia, patients should continue using contraception. Because compliance to having post-vasectomy semen analysis is so low, I offer patients the option of at home testing kits although preliminary data does not show this to improve compliance overly much [4].

6.7 Vasectomy in Patients with Pre-existing Spermatocele

Spermatoceles are essentially microscopic aneurysms of the 115 μ diameter, 15ft. long epididymis (see Chap. 5). They arise from the efferent ducts and are filled with sperm. They are found in approximately 30% of all men on whom routine ultrasound is performed, a majority of which are relatively small, under 1 cm and asymptomatic. If a man is coming for vasectomy, however, obstruction of the vas will increase the pressure in the epididymis and often cause the spermatocele to enlarge. Patients should be carefully examined pre-vasectomy, their epididymides should be palpated after the testis is warmed with a heating pad, and if a spermatocele is suspected, transilluminate the epididymis with a bright light. If it transilluminates, you know it is cystic. If it is at the caput of the epididymis as opposed to the cauda, it is almost certainly a spermatocele. Patients should be warned that if they have a small one, it could enlarge and may eventually require removal. If a patient presents with a significant spermatocele at the time of vasectomy consultation, meaning more than 2.5 cm in diameter, I would often recommend that the spermatocele be microsurgically removed at the time of the vasectomy to avoid that complication. At the very least, all patients with spermatoceles should be warned that doing a vasectomy has a significant risk of the spermatocele increasing in size, becoming symptomatic and ultimately requiring surgery.

6.8 Post-vasectomy Pain

Overall rates of post-vasectomy pain have been reported in up to 15% of all men, with 24% in men who have undergone non-no-scalpel technique and 7% in no-scalpel technique [5]. This is defined as chronic pain lasting more than 3 months after the vasectomy. With the no-scalpel vasectomy, the vas is cleanly plucked out of its sheath, preserving the vasal veins, vasal artery, which also supplies significant blood to the testicle, and the vasal nerves. By excluding the vasal nerves with the no-scalpel vasectomy, I believe this is the reason that I have been able to avoid a single case of chronic post-vasectomy pain after performing more than 4000 no-scalpel vasectomies.

References

1. Li S, et al. The no-scalpel vasectomy. J Urol. 1991;145:341–4.
2. Monoski M, et al. No-scalpel, no-needle vasectomy. Urology. 2006;68:9–14.
3. Lee R, Li P, Goldstein M. Simultaneous vasectomy and varicocelectomy: indications and technique. Urology. 2007;70:362–5.
4. Bradshaw A, et al. Poor compliance with postvasectomy semen testing: analysis of factors and barriers. Urology. 2020;136:146–51.
5. Auyeung AB, et al. Incidence of post-vasectomy pain: systematic review and meta-analysis. Int J Environ Res Public Health. 2020;17:1788.
6. Chiles KA, Goldstein M. No-scalpel vasectomy. In: Mulhall J, Jenkins L, editors. Atlas of office based andrology procedures. Cham: Springer; 2017. https://doi.org/10.1007/978-3-319-42178-0_8.

Microsurgical Reconstruction: Decision-Making

7

7.1 Introduction

The most common causes of vasal and epididymal obstructions are vasectomy and iatrogenic injury from previous scrotal/inguinal surgeries, particularly those performed in childhood, with an incidence of vasal obstruction due to iatrogenic injury in up to 26.7% of patients with a history of childhood hernia repair [1–3]. Obstruction of the epididymis can occur as a result of increased epididymal intratubular pressure from an extended time interval after vasal obstruction. In more than 50% of men with obstructive intervals exceeding 15 years after vasectomy, the build-up of pressure in the epididymis resulting in microscopic epididymal tubule rupture with sperm leakage has occurred on at least one side, causing epididymal sperm granuloma, resulting in epididymal obstruction. Iatrogenic epididymal obstruction can be caused by hydrocelectomy, spermatocelectomy, and inadvertent biopsy of the epididymis during attempted testis biopsy [4, 5]. Epididymitis, prostatitis, seminal vesiculitis, or urethritis may lead to male excurrent ductal obstruction. Ejaculatory duct obstruction (EDO) can result from straddle injury trauma, multiple transrectal prostate biopsies, surgery such as transurethral resection of the prostate in adults, or posterior urethral valves in children, infection, or congenital Mullerian duct cysts.

Microsurgical reconstruction remains the safest and most cost-effective treatment option for obstructive azoospermia [6–9], especially for couples who wish to avoid IVF/ICSI. It can allow natural conception, or less advanced ART such as IUI.

The lumen of the vas deferens and epididymal tubule are approximately 0.3 mm and 0.2 mm in diameter, respectively, and, therefore, precise microsurgical technique is the most important factor in the success of reconstruction as defined by return of sperm to the ejaculate. With recent improvements in microsurgical techniques, the success rate for return of sperm to the ejaculate with vasovasostomy is 99.5% in the most experienced hands [10–14], and between 48% and 84% for microsurgical vasoepididymostomy [11, 15–19]. Many patient-related factors, such as time interval since vasectomy, sperm granuloma at the site of anastomosis [20], antisperm antibodies [21], and gross appearance of the vasal fluid [22], are of prognostic value in determining the outcome of reconstruction. The age of the female partner is also critically important [5]. Most importantly, the surgeon's skill, reconstructive technique, and experience have a significant impact on surgical outcomes.

7.2 Intraoperative Evaluation of Vasal Fluid

The gross appearance of vasal fluid commonly correlates with the microscopic findings. Table 7.1 summarizes this correlation and help surgeons decide what operation to perform. The presence of copious crystal-clear fluid is a good prognostic sign even though sperm are usually not found

Table 7.1 Surgical recommendations based on gross appearance of vasal fluid and microscopic findings

Appearance of vasal fluid	Intraoperative evaluation of aspirate	Recommended surgical procedure
Copious, crystal clear, watery	No sperm	Vasovasostomy
Copious, cloudy thin, water soluble	Sperm with tails	Vasovasostomy
Copious, creamy yellow, water insoluble	Many sperm heads, occasional sperm with short tails	Vasovasostomy
Copious, thick white toothpaste-like, water insoluble	No sperm	Vasoepididymostomy
Scant white thin fluid	No sperm	Vasoepididymostomy
Scant fluid, no granuloma at vasectomy site	No sperm	Vasoepididymostomy
Scant fluid, granuloma present at vasectomy site	Barbotage fluid reveals sperm	Vasovasostomy

M. Goldstein, *Atlas of Male Infertility Microsurgery*, https://doi.org/10.1007/978-3-031-31601-2_7

microscopically. A vasovasostomy is indicated and the prognosis for return of sperm is over 95%. Thin cloudy fluid invariably reveals the presence of sperm microscopically and a vasovasostomy is always indicated. Creamy yellow fluid is associated with the presence of sperm parts, short-tailed sperm, and macrophages. A vasovasostomy is performed with a good prognosis for return of motile sperm. Thick, white toothpaste-like fluid indicates epididymal obstruction. Microscopic examination generally reveals a complete absence of sperm. In this setting, vasoepididymostomy is necessary. The presence of a sperm granuloma at the vasectomy site is an excellent prognostic sign. Although the testicular side lumen is often small and contains scant or no fluid, barbotage of the testicular end of the vas invariably reveals the presence of sperm and a vasovasostomy is indicated.

7.3 Vasotomy and Vasogram

Evaluation of vasal fluid (Table 7.1), in conjunction with vasography, is essential in determining the appropriate reconstruction method [23]. Most of this information has been derived from vasectomy reversal studies. In men with probable obstructive azoospermia, not caused by vasectomy, vasography with radiographic contrast media and intraoperative X-ray is rarely indicated, even in these men. Vasography should not be done at the time of testicular biopsy unless wet prep biopsy reveals sperm with tails and immediate reconstruction is undertaken. If performed carelessly, vasography can cause stricture, or even obstruction, at the vasography site, which can complicate subsequent reconstruction efforts. In addition, because most non-vasectomy-related obstructions are epididymal, vasography is of no value in making the diagnosis.

Vasography is indicated in patients in whom the diagnosis of obstructive azoospermia is fairly certain as suggested by a normal serum FSH, normal testis volume, a highly positive serum antisperm antibody assay [24], especially combined with a history of inguinal hernia repair, hydrocelectomy or epididymitis, as well as at least one palpable vas deferens. Of course, if a prior testicular biopsy reveals normal spermatogenesis, obstruction is certain. Vasography, if necessary, should be performed at the time of scrotal exploration and definitive repair of obstruction. In these men, in the presence of normal spermatogenesis, absence of sperm in the vasal fluid indicates epididymal obstruction. Vasography is done in this case with either saline or methylene blue or indigo carmine to confirm patency of the abdominal side vas prior to vasoepididymostomy. When copious sperm or sperm parts are found in the vasal fluid, the epididymis is not obstructed and vasography is indicated. Finally, when copious, thick, white fluid with no sperm is found in a dilated vas, this could indicate vasal and/or ejaculatory duct obstruction, in addition to epididymal obstruction. In these cases, simultaneous vasoepididymostomy and repair of inguinal vasal or ejaculatory duct obstruction is never successful and sperm retrieval for IVF/ICSI is indicated.

If the site of obstruction is unknown, and there is no previous inguinal incision, the testis is delivered through a high vertical scrotal incision. The vas deferens is identified and isolated at the junction of the straight and convoluted portions of the vas deferens. Using an operating microscope and 10-power magnification, the vasal sheath is vertically incised and the vasal vessels are carefully preserved.

7.4 Technique of Vasography and Interpretation of Findings

A clean segment of bare vas is delivered and a straight clamp is placed beneath the vas to act as a platform. Under 25-power magnification, a microknife is used to hemi-transect the vas until the lumen is revealed (Fig. 7.1). Any fluid exuding from the lumen is placed on a slide, mixed with a drop of saline, and sealed with a coverslip for microscopic examination. If the vasal fluid is devoid of sperm, epididymal obstruction is present. The seminal vesicle end of the vas is then cannulated with a 24-gauge angiocatheter sheath and is injected with saline to confirm patency (Fig. 7.2). If the saline passes easily, formal vasography is not necessary. If further proof of patency of the vas deferens is desired, dilute methylene blue or indigo carmine may be injected and the bladder catheterized. The presence of blue dye in the urine confirms patency of the vas. If saline does not inject, especially if inguinal scars are present, a 2-0 proline suture is passed and a clamp placed on it where it stops. The length of proline from the clamp to the point it stops is marked on the skin, indicating the location of obstruction. If it passes much further that suggests retroperitoneal obstruction.

If a large amount of fluid is found in the vasal lumen, and microscopic examination reveals the presence of sperm, obstruction toward the seminal vesicle end of the vas is likely. In these cases, the vas is usually markedly dilated and a No. 3 whistle tip ureteral catheter can be gently passed toward the seminal vesicle end of the vas. A 16-French balloon is filled with 5 mL of air. Applying gentle traction to the balloon prior to vasography prevents reflux of contrast material into the bladder from the obscuring detail (Fig. 7.3) and identifies the location of the bladder neck relative to any obstruction. After both vasa and been cannulated with three French ureteral catheters, simultaneous vasograms are performed with the injection of 50% water-soluble contrast media into both vasa (Fig. 7.4). If vasography reveals obstruction at the site of the ejaculatory ducts (Fig. 7.5), methylene blue is injected into both vasa to facilitate a trans-

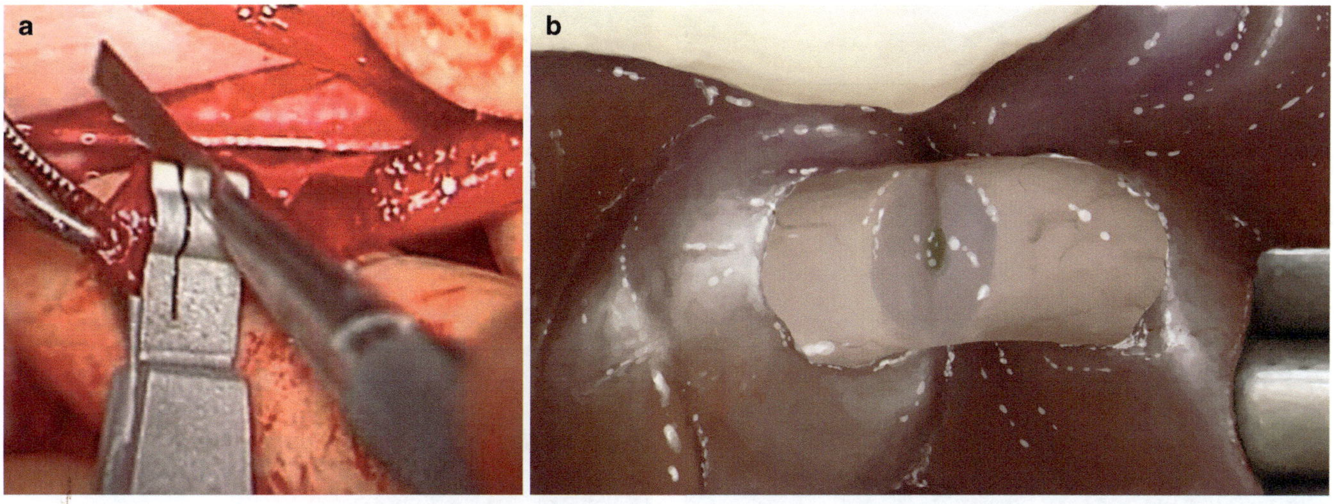

Fig. 7.1 (**a**, **b**) A microknife is used to hemi-transect the vas until the lumen is revealed

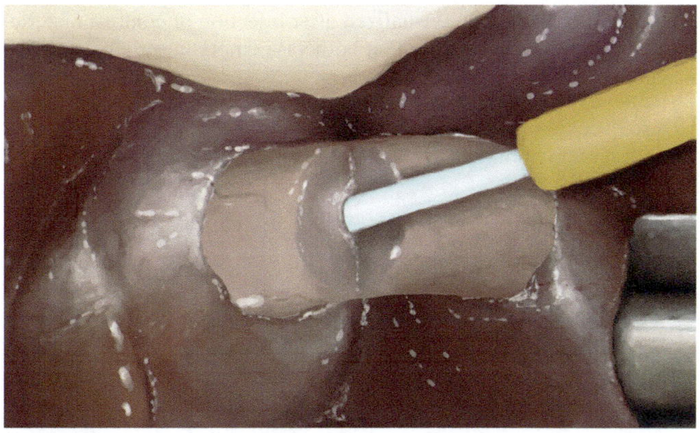

Fig. 7.2 The seminal vesicle end of the vas is then cannulated with a 24-gauge angiocatheter sheath and is injected with saline to confirm patency

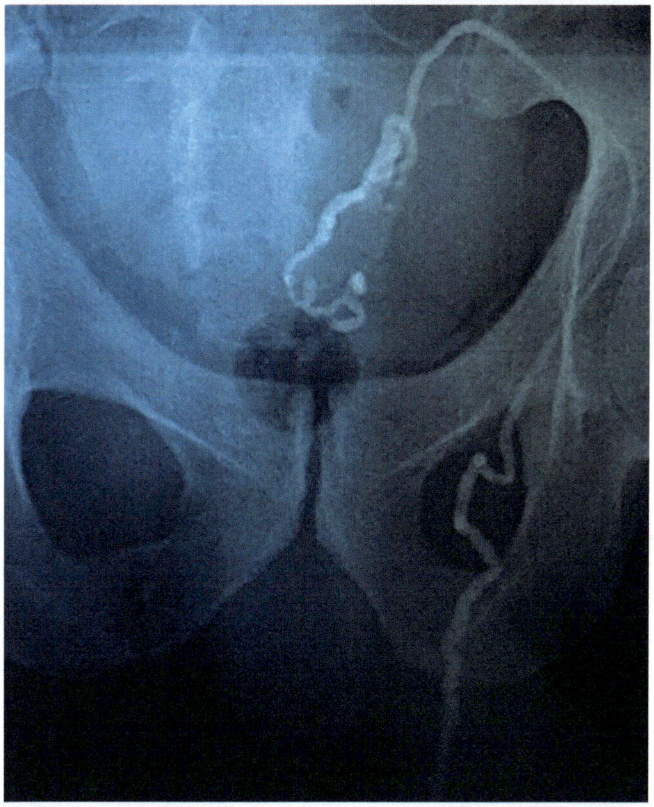

Fig. 7.3 A 16-French balloon is filled with 5 mL of air. Applying gentle traction to the balloon prior to vasography prevents reflux of contrast material into the bladder from the obscuring detail

urethral resection of the ejaculatory ducts (TUR-ED). If both vasa are visualized after injection of contrast material into only one vas (Fig. 7.6), it indicates that both vasa empty into a single cavity, usually a midline Müllerian duct cyst.

Vasography may reveal that the vas deferens blindly ends far away from the ejaculatory ducts (congenital bilateral partial absence of the vas deferens). If this is found bilaterally (Fig. 7.7), no further reconstructive surgery is indicated, and vasal/epididymal/testicular sperm is retrieved and cryopreserved for IVF/ICSI. If vasography reveals obstruction in the inguinal region (Fig. 7.8), either inguinal vasovasostomy or crossed transeptal vasovasostomy may be performed. Vasography sites are carefully closed with microsurgical technique using 10-0 monofilament nylon for the mucosa and 9-0 for the muscularis and adventitia. If the vasal fluid reveals no sperm, and injection of the seminal vesicle end of the vas confirms its patency, then the vas is completely transected and the end is prepared for vasoepididymostomy. If the vasal fluid reveals many sperm and vasography is normal, either lack of emission or aperistalsis of the vas [25] is the cause of azoospermia and electroejaculation and/or sperm retrieval is performed.

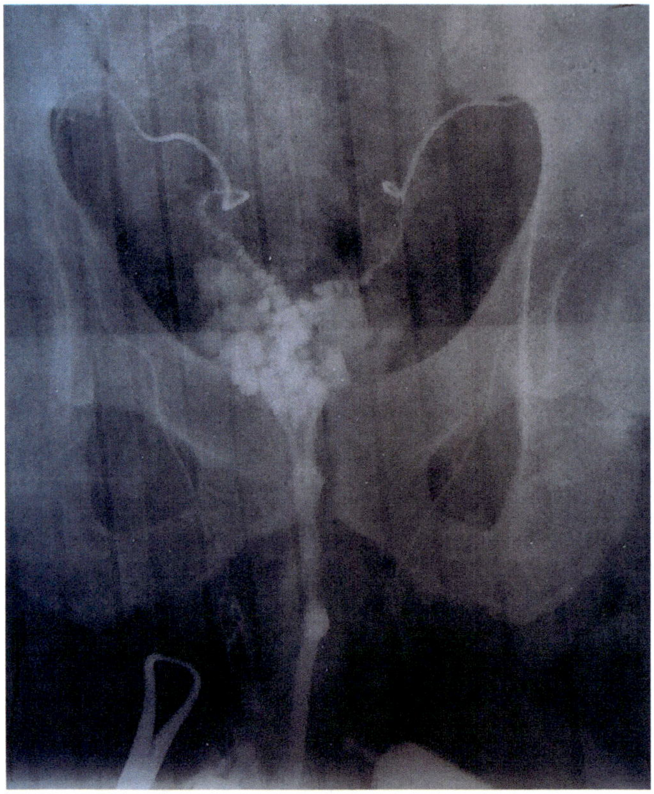

Fig. 7.4 Simultaneous vasograms are performed with the injection of 50% water-soluble contrast media into both vasa

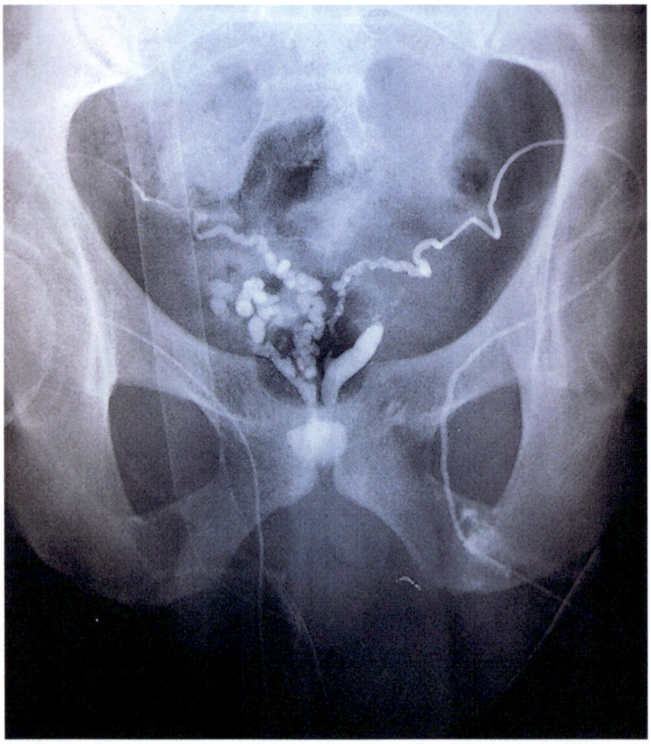

Fig. 7.5 If vasography reveals obstruction at the site of the ejaculatory ducts, methylene blue is injected into both vasa to facilitate a transurethral resection of the ejaculatory ducts (TUR-ED)

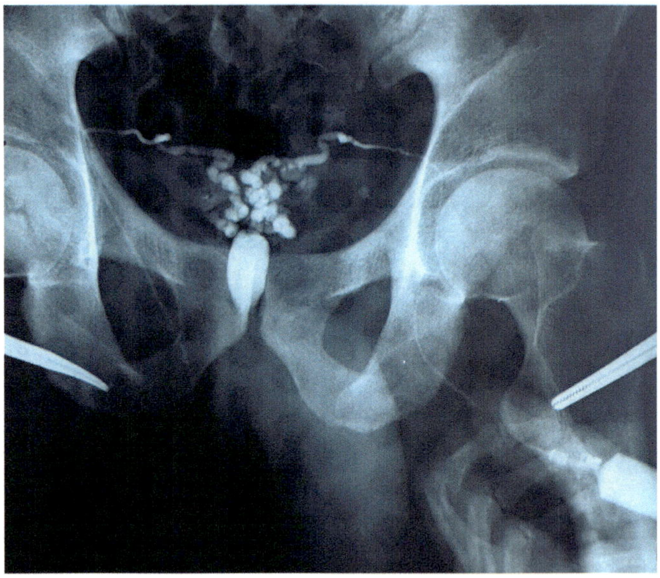

Fig. 7.6 If both vasa are visualized after injection of contrast material into only one vas, it indicates that both vasa empty into a single cavity, usually a midline Müllerian duct cyst

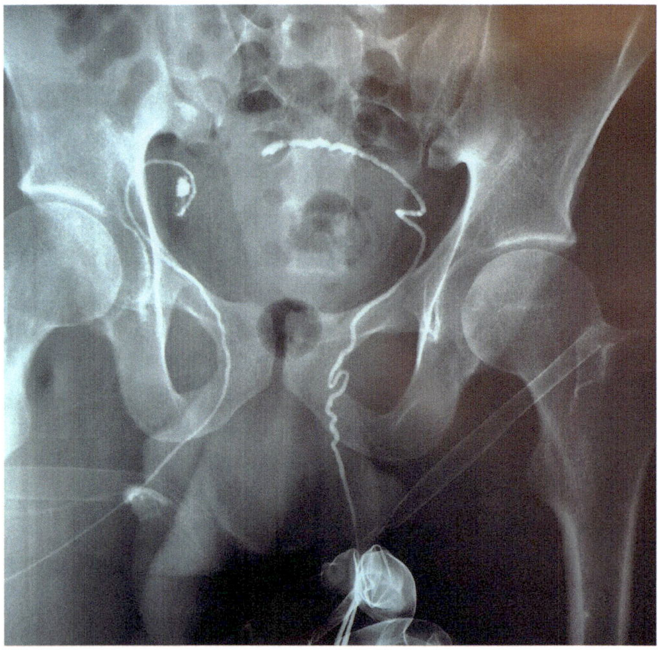

Fig. 7.7 Vasography may reveal that the vas deferens blindly ends far away from the ejaculatory ducts (congenital bilateral partial absence of the vas deferens). If this is found bilaterally, no further reconstructive surgery is indicated

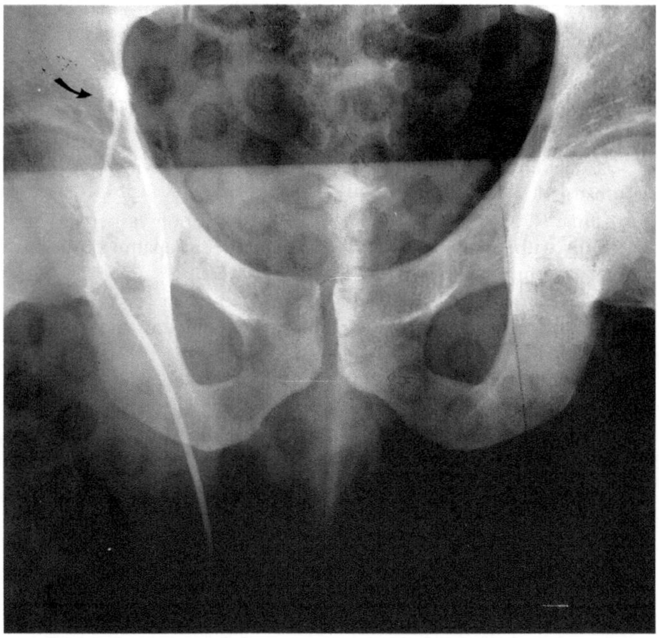

Fig. 7.8 If vasography reveals obstruction in the inguinal region, either inguinal vasovasostomy or crossed transeptal vasovasostomy may be performed

7.5 Contrast Agents for Vasography

Ringer's lactate or normal saline should be used first. If the fluid injects easily toward the seminal vesicle end of the vas, contrast vasography is unnecessary. For confirmation of patency, or if injection of saline requires undue pressure, methylene blue or indigo carmine can be injected and the bladder catheterized. The presence of dye in the bladder indicates patency. The inability to inject requires formal vasography with 50% dilated water-soluble contrast material. If vasography reveals ejaculatory duct obstruction, methylene blue is instilled to assist in TUR-ed. A 2-0 nylon or proline suture may be passed to localize inguinal obstruction, but when groin scars are present, exploration is best done through the old scar. This approach will usually lead to the inguinal obstruction and obviate the need for a separate vasotomy or vasogram.

7.6 Complications of Vasography

Stricture: Multiple attempts at percutaneous vasography using sharp needles can result in stricture or obstruction at the vasography site. Careless or crude closure of a vasotomy can also result in stricture and obstruction. Non-water-soluble contrast agents may also result in stricture and should not be employed for vasography.

Injury to the vasal blood supply: If the vasal blood supply is injured at the site of vasography, vasovasostomy proximal to the vasography site may result in ischemia, necrosis, and obstruction of the intervening segment of the vas.

Hematoma: Bipolar cautery should be used for meticulous hemostasis at the time of vasostomy to prevent hematoma in the perivasal sheath.

Sperm granuloma: Leaky closure of a vasography site may lead to the development of a sperm granuloma, which can result in stricture or obstruction of the vas. The microsurgical technique for closure of vasography sites is identical to that employed for vasovasostomy described later in Chap. 8.

7.7 Transrectal Vasography and Seminal Vesiculography

If transrectal ultrasonographic study reveals markedly dilated seminal vesicles or a midline cyst, or both, in a man with obstructive azoospermia, transrectal aspiration followed by instillation of methylene blue mixed with contrast agent is a useful diagnostic and potentially therapeutic maneuver.

The same bowel preparation procedure and antibiotic coverage used for transrectal prostate biopsy is employed. The fine-needle aspirate is examined for sperm. If sperm are present, t means at least one vas and epididymis are unobstructed. Dilution of 0.5 mL of methylene blue is accomplished with 1.5 mL of 50% water-soluble contrast. If a flat plate radiograph reveals a potentially resectable lesion, a TUR-ED is performed (Chap. 12). Visualization of methylene blue effluxing from the ejaculatory ducts or unroofed cyst confirms the adequacy of the resection.

The aspirated sperm are analyzed and then cryopreserved for possible future IVF/ICSI in case the surgery fails. If no sperm are found in the aspirated fluid, a secondary epididymal obstruction is present. The tunica vaginalis is opened and the epididymis is inspected under the operating microscope. If there is clear evidence of epididymal obstruction (i.e., if an epididymal sperm granuloma is present and there is a clear line of demarcation—dilated and indurated above, soft and collapsed below), vasoepididymostomy is performed after the TUR-ED.

This technique obviates the need for formal open scrotal vasography in men with transrectally accessible lesions. If sperm are found in the aspirate, a TUR-ED may immediately be undertaken without violating the scrotum. Sperm-laden aspirates may be cryopreserved for future IVF with ICSI if surgery fails.

Tips

- For vasography, make sure not to completely transect the vas deferens.
- Gently dilate and gently inject saline and/or contrast agent.

References

1. Matsuda T. Diagnosis and treatment of post-herniorrhaphy vas deferens obstruction. Int J Urol. 2000;7:S35–8.
2. Chen X, et al. Clinical features and therapeutic strategies of obstructive azoospermia in patients treated by bilateral inguinal hernia repair in childhood. Asian J Androl. 2014;16:745–8.
3. Sheynkin Y, et al. Microsurgical repair of iatrogenic injury to the vas deferens. J Urol. 1998;159:139–41.
4. Hopps CV, Goldstein M. Microsurgical reconstruction of iatrogenic injuries to the epididymis from hydrocelectomy. J Urol. 2006;176:2077–80.
5. Fuchs E, Burt R. Vasectomy reversal performed 15 years or more after vasectomy: correlation of pregnancy outcome with partner age and with pregnancy results of in vitro fertilization with intracytoplasmic sperm injection. Fertil Steril. 2002;77:516–9.
6. Lee RK, et al. Reassessing reconstruction in the management of obstructive azoospermia: reconstruction or sperm acquisition? Urol Clin N Am. 2008;35:289–301.
7. Donovan J, et al. Comparison of microscopic epididymal sperm aspiration and intracytoplasmic sperm injection/in-vitro fertilization with repeat microscopic reconstruction following vasectomy: is second attempt vas reversal worth the effort? Hum Reprod. 1998;13(2):387–93.
8. Pavlovich C, Schlegel P. Fertility options after vasectomy: a cost-effective analysis. Fertil Steril. 1997;67:133–41.
9. Kolettis O, Thomas A. Vasoepididymostomy for vasectomy reversal: a critical analysis in the era of intracytoplasmic sperm injection. J Urol. 1997;158:467–70.
10. Harrel L, et al. Outcomes of microsurgical vasovasostomy for vasectomy reversal: a meta-analysis and systematic review. Urology. 2015;85(4):819–25.
11. Matthews G, Schlegel P, Goldstein M. Patency following microsurgical vasoepididymostomy and vasovasostomy: temporal considerations. J Urol. 1995;154(6):2070–3.
12. Goldstein M, Li P, Matthews G. Microsurgical vasovasostomy: the microdot technique of precision suture placement. J Urol. 1998;159(1):188–90.
13. Belker A, et al. Results of 1469 microsurgical vasectomy reversals by the vasovasostomy study group. J Urol. 1991;145(3):505–11.
14. Silber S. Microscopic vasectomy reversal. Fertil Steril. 1977;28(11):1191–202.
15. Peng J, et al. Pregnancy and live birth rates after microsurgical vasoepididymostomy for azoospermic patients with epididymal obstruction. Hum Reprod. 2017;32(2):284–9.
16. Kumar R, Mukherjee S, Gupta N. Intussusception vasoepididymostomy with longitudinal suture placement for idiopathic obstructive azoospermia. J Urol. 2010;183(4):1489–92.
17. Chan P, Brandell R, Goldstein M. Prospective analysis of outcomes after microsurgical intussusception vaso-epididymostomy. BJU Int. 2005;96(4):598–601.
18. Silber S. Results of microsurgical vasoepididymostomy: role of epididymis in sperm maturation. Hum Reprod. 1989;4:298–303.
19. Schiff J, et al. Outcome and late failures compared in 4 techniques of microsurgical vaso-epididymostomy in 153 consecutive men. J Urol. 2005;174:651–5.
20. Boorjian S, Lipkin M, Goldstein M. The impact of obstructive interval and sperm granuloma on outcome of vasectomy reversal. J Urol. 2004;171:304–6.
21. Meinertz H, et al. Antisperm antibodies and fertility after vasovasostomy: a follow-up study of 216 men. Fertil Steril. 1990;54(2):315–21.
22. Goldstein M. Surgical management of male infertility. In: Partin A, et al., editors. Campbell Walsh Wein urology. Amsterdam: Elsevier; 2020.
23. Wosnitzer M, Goldstein M. Obstructive azoospermia. In: Neiderberger CS, editor. Current management of male infertility. Philadelphia, PA: Elsevier; 2014. p. 83–95.
24. Lee RK, et al. Value of serum antisperm antibodies in diagnosing obstructive azoospermia. J Urol. 2009;181:264–9.
25. Tiffany P, Goldstein M. Aperistalsis of the vas deferens corrected with administration of ephedrine. J Urol. 1985;133:1060–1.

8 Microsurgical Vasovasostomy

There are few procedures where the outcomes are so dependent on technical perfection. Keys to success are: (1) cut back until you find good vasal blood supply; (2) perfect mucosal approximation; and (3) three to four layers to remove all tension from the anastomosis.

Vasectomy is the contraceptive method of choice for 42–60 million men worldwide, with approximately 500,000 men undergoing the procedure in North America each year [1, 2]. Before undergoing the vasectomy, the patient should receive counseling regarding the permanency of the procedure and be offered the option of sperm banking. Patients should also be counselled that successful reversal of elective sterilization is not guaranteed. There exists some controversy regarding the impact of obstructive interval on the outcome of vasectomy reversal. A 2004 series of 213 patients from a single surgeon performing microsurgical vasectomy reversals concluded that while there was no impact on patency rates, but an obstructive interval of over 15 years negatively impacted pregnancy rates [3]. The older study by the Vasovasostomy Study Group found a decreased likelihood of patency with increasing obstructive interval [4]. Regardless of obstructive interval, the best predictor of successful vasectomy reversal of the presence of complete (motile or immotile) sperm or sperm with short tails or abundant sperm heads, some with identifiable acrosomes, in the vasal fluid at the time of the procedure [5, 6]. Despite pre-operative counseling, surveys suggest that 2–6% of vasectomized men will ultimately seek vasectomy reversal, and some series have shown this number can be as high as 20%, although not all men who are evaluated for reversal proceed with the procedure, mainly due to financial constraints [7].

8.1 Microdot Multi-Layer Technique

The microdot technique is the first step in my multi-layer technique and is designed to accurately approximate the vasal mucosa. I developed this technique as a means of improving the suture placement by the exact mapping of each planned suture. While a one-layer technique is simpler, quicker and requires less microsurgical training, it does not allow as precise mucosa-to-mucosa approximation when luminal diameters are very disparate [8]. With long obstructive intervals, especially in the absence of a sperm granuloma, discrepancies of 3:1 or even 5:1 are common. Since the outer diameter of the vas is unchanged with long obstructive intervals, when the testicular lumen is enlarged, it is due to a loss of muscle, so the muscle layer on the testicular end is much thinner than the abdominal end and a single-layer technique results in "shelving" where the mucosal lumen does not line up edge-to-edge. Employing a multi-layer technique in which the mucosa is first reapproximated, followed by the muscle, adventitia, and sheath requires greater microsurgical training but results in a more watertight anastomosis [9]. When sperm are found in the fluid emanating from the testicular end of the vas, the patency rate of this technique for return of sperm to the ejaculate is 89.4–99.5%, and the pregnancy rate with partners under the age of 36 without female factor, for patients undergoing this procedure is 73% [10].

8.1.1 The Microdot Method Separates the Planning from Suture Placement

Much as an architect prepares blueprints before the contractor constructs a bridge, the planning of suture placement is critical to a successful surgical outcome. This painstaking planning allows the surgeon to focus on one task at the time of suture placement. In addition, the discrepancy in diameter between the testicular vasal lumen and the abdominal (seminal vesicle) end of the vas is typically 2:1–3:1. Careful, even spacing of the sutures minimizes luminal discrepancy and limits "dog-ears" and leaks, thus decreasing the risk of post-operative stricture, granuloma formation, and reconstructive failure [9].

M. Goldstein, *Atlas of Male Infertility Microsurgery*, https://doi.org/10.1007/978-3-031-31601-2_8

8.2 Technique

A micro-tip surgical skin marking pen (Devon™, Model # 31145942) is used to map out planned needle exit points (Fig. 8.1). All mucosal sutures are placed with double-armed sutures so that they are all placed from the inside out (Fig. 8.2). This way no instruments need to be introduced into the mucosa to grab the needle. This minimizes instrumentation of the mucosa. After placing the first three mucosal sutures, one should clearly see a "three-string guitar" appearance of the sutures, guaranteeing that the sutures are not crossed (Fig. 8.3). Exactly six monofilament double-armed 10-0 nylon mucosal sutures (first layer) are used for every anastomosis (Fig. 8.4). After completion of the mucosal layer, six 9-0 deep muscularis sutures are placed exactly in between each mucosal suture, just superficial to, but not penetrating, the mucosa (second layer) (Fig. 8.5). Six additional 9-0 nylon interrupted sutures are then placed between each muscular suture (third layer). Finally, six 8-0 nylon sutures are placed approximating the adventitia of the vas deferens (Fig. 8.6). All anastomoses consist of four layers of six sutures, for a total of 24 sutures. The dartos layer is approximated with interrupted 4-0 absorbable sutures and the skin with subcuticular sutures of a 5-0 monofilament absorbable suture.

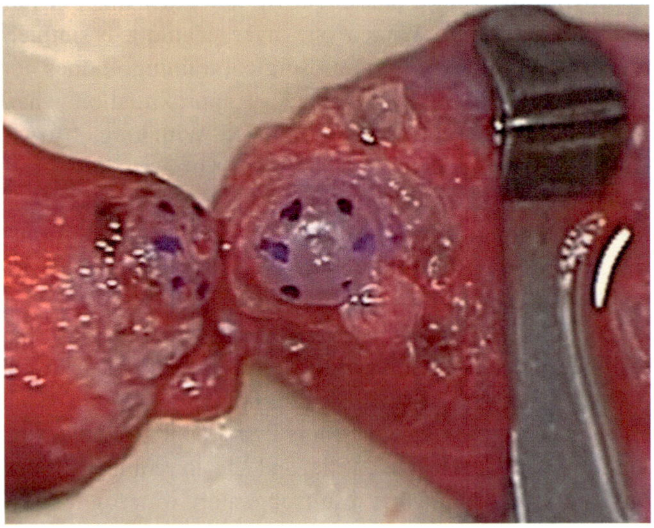

Fig. 8.1 A micro-tip surgical skin marking pen (Devon™, Model # 31145942) is used to map out planned needle exit points

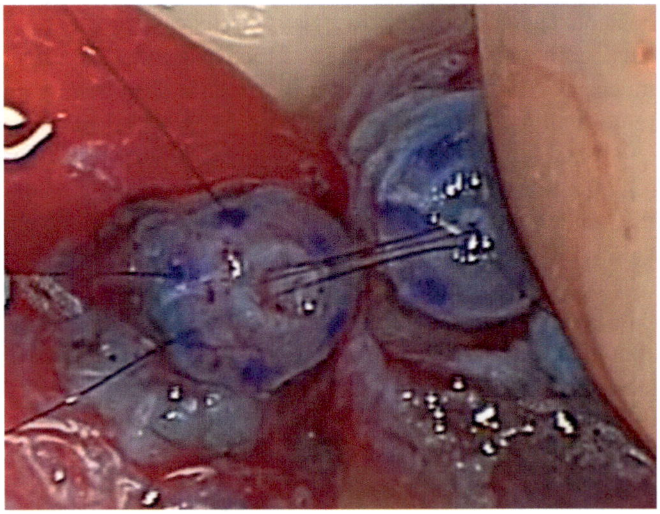

Fig. 8.3 After placing the first 3 mucosal sutures, one should clearly see a "three-string guitar" appearance of the sutures, guaranteeing that the sutures are not crossed

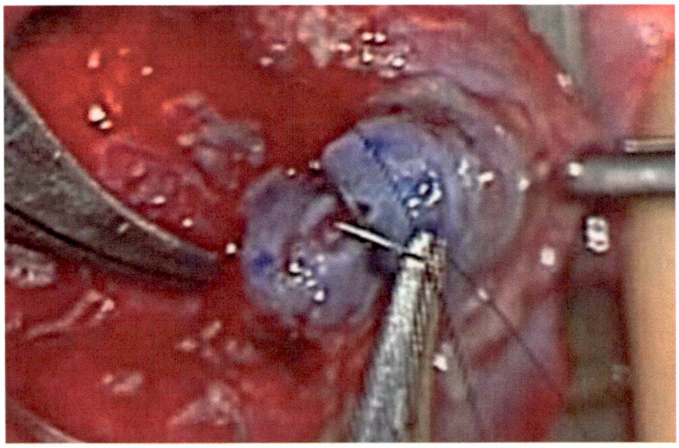

Fig. 8.2 All mucosal sutures are placed with double-armed sutures so that they are all placed from the inside out

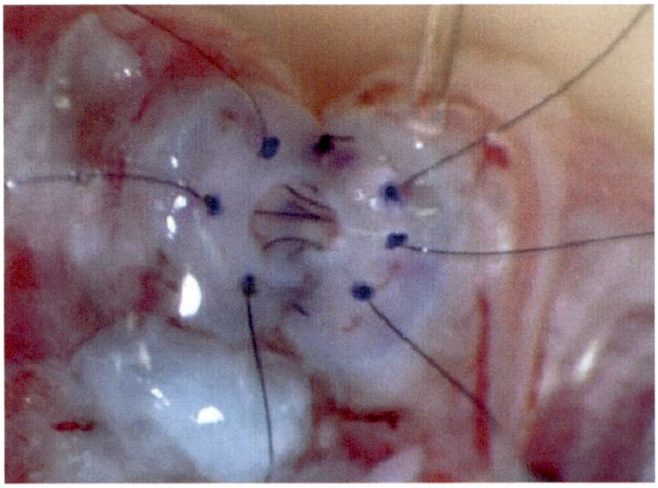

Fig. 8.4 Appearance just prior to tying the final three 10-0 mucosal sutures. (*From* Kolettis and Goldstein [17]; *with permission*)

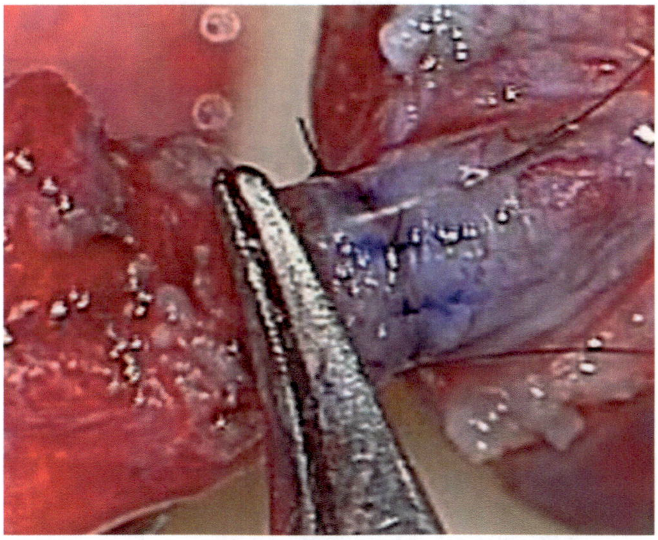

Fig. 8.5 Six additional 9-0 nylon interrupted sutures are then placed between each muscular suture (second layer)

8.3 Inguinal Obstruction

If vasography reveals obstruction in the inguinal region, either inguinal vasovasostomy or, ideally, crossed transeptal vasovasostomy, using the contralateral unobstructed vas may be performed.

8.4 Crossed Vasovasostomy

A crossed vasovasostomy is indicated when there is either a unilateral inguinal obstruction of the vas deferens associated with an atrophic testis on the contralateral side, or there is obstruction or aplasia of the inguinal vas or ejaculatory duct on one side and epididymal obstruction on the contralateral side. **It is preferable to perform one anastomosis with a high probability of success (vasovasostomy) than two operations with a much lower chance of success**, such as a vasoepididymostomy with a contralateral transurethral resection of the ejaculatory ducts.

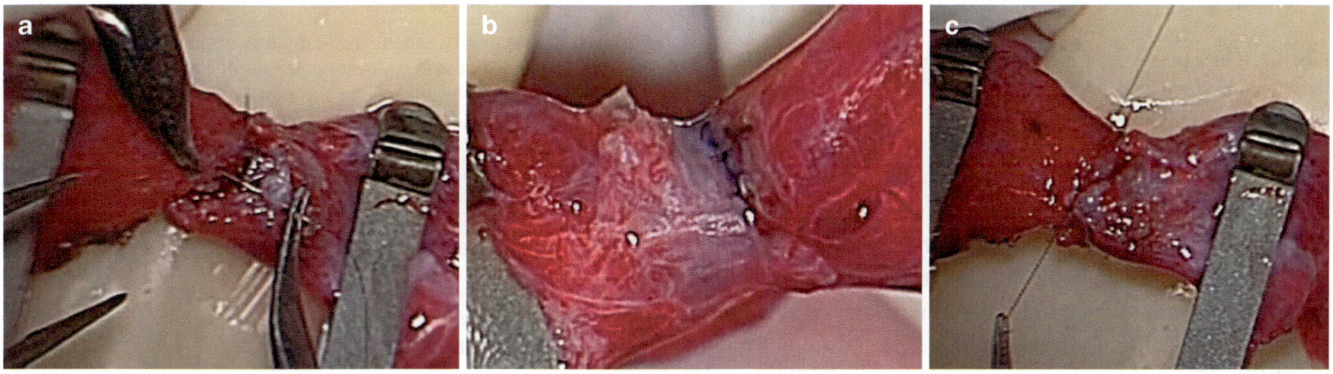

Fig. 8.6 (**a**, **b**) Finally, six 8-0 nylon sutures are placed through the adventitia of the vas deferens placed exactly between the six sutures from the preceding layer. (**c**) Appearance of the adventitia just after tying the first adventitial suture

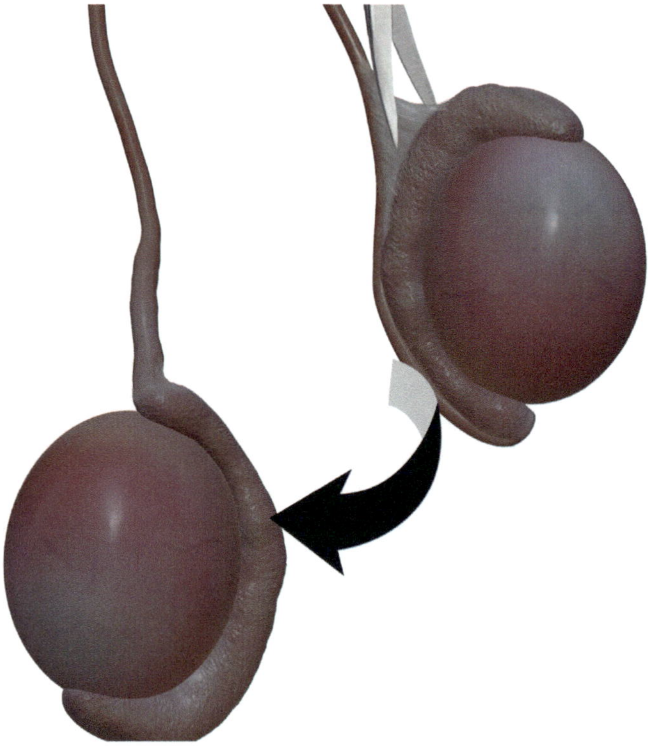

Fig. 8.7 Once presence of sperm or sperm parts in the testicular end of the lumen is confirmed, the testicular end of the vas is crossed through a capacious opening made in the scrotal septum

The procedure begins by first transecting the vas attached to the atrophic testis at the junction of its straight and convoluted portion and confirming its patency with a Ringer's or indigo carmine vasogram. The contralateral vas from the normal testis is dissected to the vasotomy site, or, if inguinal obstruction is certain, after sampling of the testicular and of vasal fluid to confirm the presence of sperm. The testicular end of the vas is transected as high up as possible with a right-angle clamp. Once presence of sperm or sperm parts in the testicular end of the lumen is confirmed, the testicular end of the vas is crossed through a capacious opening made in the scrotal septum (Fig. 8.7). A microsurgical vasovasostomy, as described above, is then performed. This procedure is much easier than an inguinal vasovasostomy, which requires finding both ends of the vas within the dense scar tissue from previous inguinal surgery. The outcomes are almost always as good as ipsilateral vasovasostomy [11].

8.5 Transposition of the Testis

Occasionally when vasal length is critically short, a tension-free crossed anastomosis can best be accomplished by testicular transposition. The testis easily passes through a generous opening in the septum to sit nicely in the contralateral scrotal compartment next to the adjacent testis (Fig. 8.8).

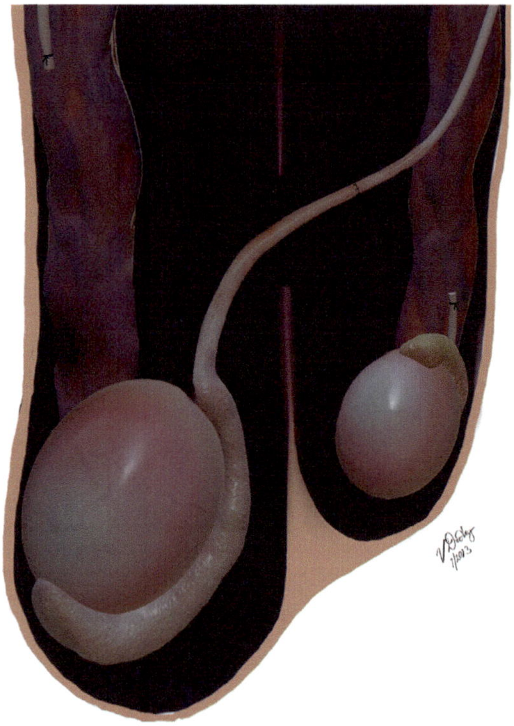

Fig. 8.8 Occasionally, when vasal length is critically short, a tension-free crossed anastomosis can best be accomplished by testicular transposition. The testis easily passes through a generous opening in the septum to sit nicely in the contralateral scrotal compartment next to the adjacent testis

8.6 Inguinal Vasovasostomy

Mesh used during bilateral inguinal hernia repair is associated with iatrogenic obstructive azoospermia in at least 0.1% of repairs [12, 13]. The obstruction may occur at the internal inguinal ring, making vasovasostomy challenging. In these cases, laparoscopic mobilization of the retroperitoneal vas deferens can facilitate the vasovasostomy, but although I have had initial patency, they have all shut down and no live births have ever been reported. In these cases, it is more prudent to just perform sperm retrieval for use in IVF/ICSI.

Patients with suspected iatrogenic obstructive azoospermia should first undergo microsurgical vasotomies, and vasograms to confirm bilateral inguinal obstruction at the level of the internal inguinal ring (see Fig. 7.8). Inguinal exploration directly through the hernia scars usually leads to the obstructed vas. There is always a bed of scar from the testicular end that will lead to the abdominal side. Vasovasostomy is then performed as described above.

8.7 Simultaneous Varicocelectomy and Vasovasostomy: Caveat Emptor

When men presenting for vasovasostomy or vasoepididymostomy are found to have significant varicoceles on physical examination, it is tempting to repair of the varicoceles at the same time. I prefer to avoid this. When varicocelectomy is properly performed, all spermatic veins are ligated and the only remaining avenues for testicular venous return are the vasal veins. In men who have undergone vasectomy and are presenting for reversal, the vasal veins are likely to be compromised from either the original vasectomy or the reversal itself. Furthermore, the integrity of the vasal artery in those men is also likely to be compromised. Varicocelectomy in such men requires preservation of the testicular artery as the primary remaining testicular blood supply, as well as preservation of some avenue for venous return. Microsurgical varicocelectomy can ensure preservation of the testicular artery in most cases. Deliberate preservation of the cremasteric veins provides venous return. Of 407 men presenting for vasectomy reversal, 14 had large varicoceles (10 on the left; 4 that were bilateral).

Microsurgical varicocelectomy was performed at the same time as vasovasostomy. The cremasteric veins and the fine network of veins adherent to the testicular artery were left intact for venous return and to minimize the chances of injury to the testicular artery. Postoperative, 4 of 18 varicoceles recurred (22%) and two testes atrophied (11%). This experience contrasts with a recurrence rate of 0.6% and no cases of atrophy in 640 varicocelectomies performed by the author in non-vasectomized men in whom the vasal vessels were intact and the cremasteric veins and periarterial venous network were ligated.

There is debate about the safety of simultaneous varicocelectomy and vasal reconstruction. Mulhall et al. found no postoperative testicular atrophy or hydrocele formation in patients who underwent simultaneous varicocelectomy and vasovasostomy when performed by experienced microsurgeons [14]. Because of the significantly increased risk of testicular atrophy and varicocele recurrence, varicocelectomy should only be performed at the same time as vasovasostomy when the surgeon has extensive experience in microsurgery. Because of concerns regarding lack of adequate venous return, and the high venous pressure on the abdominal vas to be used for the anastomosis that would result, we do not recommend doing varicocelectomy in conjunction with vasoepididymostomy. Rather, the vasoepididymostomy should be performed first, and the quality of semen should be determined postoperatively. If necessary, varicocelectomy can safety be performed 6 months or more later, when venous and arterial channels have formed across the anastomotic line. This two-staged delayed approach has been utilized a dozen times with no incidence of atrophy or recurrence.

Interestingly, the significant increase in recurrences in our series when the cremasteric veins and periarterial venous network were left intact suggest that these veins contribute to a significant proportion of varicocele recurrences.

8.8 Simultaneous Sperm Retrieval at the Time of Vasovasostomy or Vasoepididymostomy

Anytime a vasoepididymostomy is performed, I strongly recommend simultaneous intraoperative retrieval of sperm with cryopreservation and a TUNEL assay to assess the DNA integrity. Vasoepididymostomy has an approximate 80% success rate in terms of return of sperm. Since 20% of the time the procedure will not result in return of sperm, if you have retrieved sperm intraoperatively, you will have a backup that can be used for IVF/ICSI. I would also retrieve sperm at the time of vasovasostomy if there is any doubt about the health of the vas, the blood supply to the vas, or the quality of the anastomosis, so in case there is a failure, they will already have sperm retrieved that can then be used for IVF/ICSI. In addition, the late failure rate for vasovasostomy is approximately 15%, and for vasoepididymostomy is 25% [15, 16]. This means that at 18 months post procedure, men who initially had sperm will be azoospermic. If sperm were frozen intraoperative, you will have that as a backup, although **we routinely recommend that men, once they get return of motile sperm to the ejaculate after vasovasostomy or vasoepididymostomy, that they cryopreserve those sperm** so if they if they do shut down later on, they will have sperm they can use if the quality is good for IUI, but definitely if they are alive, can be used for IVF/ICSI. If it is during a vasoepididymostomy, we recommend retrieving sperm from the tubule after it is opened, and this can be done with micropipettes as described in Chap. 10. I also recommend retrieving sperm directly from the testis via biopsy as described in Chap. 11, and this way a TUNEL assay can be done to assess the DNA integrity of all different sites from which sperm were retrieved, then we can tell the IVF doctors which is the best sperm that would result in the highest chance of live delivery after IVF/ICSI.

Tips

- Always use two hands for placing every stitch. For a righty, use your left hand to support the right hand, and vice versa if you are a lefty.
- A micro-vessel dilator is the best instrument for grabbing a very short 10-0 suture end to pull it back and avoid losing the suture.

- A micro-vessel dilator and a #5 fine-tipped jeweler's forceps combined can allow you to tie very short (1 cm length) of 10-0 suture and avoid losing the stitch.

8.9 Vasovasostomy or Vasoepididymostomy: Postoperative Care

I tell my patients that it is likely that they will have some discomfort for the first 2–3 weeks after surgery. At the time of discharge from the hospital, I prescribe pain medication, and instruct them to be careful while walking or climbing stairs, as dizziness is not unusual while taking pain medication. I also prescribe a course of Celebrex, taken the night prior to surgery and for 6 days thereafter to help reduce inflammation and decrease dependence on postoperative pain killers.

I have patients return to the office for postoperative examination 4 weeks following the procedure. At the same time, I have the patient provide a sperm sample, which I examine under a bench microscope. In the presence of sperm in the ejaculate, the patient and his partner can start attempting to conceive immediately. I typically also recommend to these patients that they cryopreserve ejaculated specimens at this time in the event of a late shutdown.

In some patients who are at high risk for stricture or failure of the anastomosis, I prescribe a course of prednisone to prevent shutdown. I start with 20 mg twice a day for days one through ten of the partner's menstrual cycle, followed by 5 mg daily for the remainder of the month. I keep the patient on this dosage for at least 6 months, or until the partner conceives. In the event after 6 months, the partner has not yet conceived, recommend the patient have an antisperm antibody assay and a complete semen analysis.

I explain that swelling and bruising of the penis and scrotum are normal and will take about 3 weeks to mostly resolve. Application of ice to the wound is the same as in the postoperative instructions for varicocelectomy. In some patients, rubber drains are left in the scrotum and will be removed the morning after the procedure. An instruction sheet for removal of the drains is given to the patient at the time of discharge; if the patient or their partner are uncomfortable performing this task, I have them return to the office the day after the procedure and either myself or my nurse can do it for them.

Patients are instructed to wear a scrotal supporter at all times, even when sleeping, for 6 weeks postoperatively. It can be removed while showering. After 6 weeks, the scrotal supporter should be worn while walking, running, engaging in sports or physical activity. The purpose of the supporter is to prevent the testes from pulling down on the reconnected ducts.

Long-term use of a scrotal supporter can lead to fungal infection. I instruct patients to ensure they completely dry themselves following showering and to make sure their scrotal supporter is clean. If fungal infection should occur, using a 50–50 combination of 1% antifungal cream and 1% hydrocortisone cream can be applied to the area three times daily.

Following vasovasostomy or vasoepididymostomy, patients are instructed to refrain from any sexual activity, including masturbation, for 4 weeks in order to avoid disturbance of the delicate anastomoses and to prevent contractions of the vas deferens. Typically, their first ejaculation following their procedure is at the time of their postoperative examination at which time I have them produce a semen sample for analysis. After this point, they may resume normal sexual activities. I have these patients repeat their semen analysis at 3 and 6 months postoperatively, and every 6 months thereafter until the patient's partner conceives.

References

1. Pile J, Barone M. Demographics of vasectomy–USA and international. Urol Clin N Am. 2009;36(3):295–305.
2. Ostrowski K, et al. Marketscan® evaluation of vasectomy trends in the United States. J Urol. 2016;195(4):e1158.
3. Boorjian S, Lipkin M, Goldstein M. The impact of obstructive interval and sperm granuloma on outcome of vasectomy reversal. J Urol. 2004;171:304–6.
4. Belker A, et al. Results of 1469 microsurgical vasectomy reversals by the vasovasostomy study group. J Urol. 1991;145(3):505–11.
5. Scovell J, et al. Association between the presence of sperm in the vasal fluid during vasectomy reversal and postoperative patency: a systematic review and meta-analysis. J Urol. 2015;85(4):809–13.
6. Goldstein M. Surgical management of male infertility. In: Partin A, et al., editors. Campbell Walsh Wein urology. Amsterdam: Elsevier; 2020.
7. Sigalos J, et al. Characteristics and motivations of men who seek vasectomy reversal. J Urol. 2017;197(4S):e1208.
8. Jarvi K, et al. Mini-incision microsurgical vasectomy reversal using no-scalpel vasectomy principles and instruments. Urology. 2008;72(4):913–5.
9. Harrel L, Hsiao W. Microsurgical vasovasostomy. Asian J Androl. 2013;15:44–8.
10. Herrel L, et al. Outcomes of microsurgical vasovasostomy for vasectomy reversal: a meta-analysis and systematic review. J Urol. 2015;85(4):819–25.
11. Sheynkin YR, et al. Microsurgical repair of iatrogenic injury to the vas deferens. J Urol. 1998;159:137–41.
12. Blouchos K, et al. Iatrogenic vas deferens injury due to inguinal hernia repair. Hellenic J Surg. 2012;84(6):356–63.
13. Schulster M, et al. Microsurgically assisted inguinal hernia repair and simultaneous male fertility procedures: rationale, technique and outcomes. J Urol. 2017;198:1168.
14. Mulhall J, et al. Simultaneous microsurgical vasal reconstruction and varicocele ligation: safety profile and outcomes. Urology. 1997;50(3):438–42.
15. Farber N, et al. The kinetics of sperm return and late failure following vasovasostomy or vasoepididymostomy: a systematic review. J Urol. 2019;201:241–50.
16. Goldstein M, Li PS, Matthews GJ. Microsurgical vasovasostomy: the microdot technique of precision suture placement. J Urol. 1998;159:188–90.
17. Kolettis PN, Goldstein M. Vasovasostomy. In: Goldstein M, Schlegel PN. Surgical and medical management of male infertility. Cambridge; Cambridge University Press; 2013.

9 Microsurgical Vasoepididymostomy

Microsurgical vasoepididymostomy is the most technically challenging microsurgery of the male reproductive system. Virtually, no other operation results are so dependent upon the surgeon's technical expertise. Surgeons who perform vasoepididymostomy, therefore, must have extensive experience in microsurgical techniques and carry out the procedure frequently. The indications for performing vasoepididymostomy at the time of vasectomy reversal, based on gross appearance of the vasal fluid [1], are reviewed in Table 7.1. Although occasional discrepancies exist between gross and microscopic findings, they correlate approximately 80% of the time. It is, however, essential to view the vasal fluid under a 400-power bench microscope, in order to determine whether to proceed with vasovasostomy or with vasoepididymostomy. For obstructive azoospermia that is not due to vasectomy or congenital absence of the vas deferens, vasoepididymostomy is indicated when the testis biopsy reveals complete spermatogenesis and vasotomy reveals the absence of sperm in the vasal lumen with a patent abdominal vas. Ultimately, success of vasoepididymostomy can be predicted based on the level of microsurgical training and skill of the surgeon, the site of the anastomosis, and the presence of sperm in the epididymal fluid [2].

9.1 Microsurgical End-to-Side Two-Suture Intussusception Vasoepididymostomy

The intussusception technique, originally known as the three-suture triangulation technique, was developed by Berger [3]. Marmar described a modified technique that consisted of two sutures with transverse double-needle placement within the epididymal tubule [4]. At Weill Cornell Medicine, my former fellow Peter Chan and I developed a two-suture longitudinal intussusception vasoepididymostomy (LIVE) approach in order to further improve the procedure [5]. With this method, four microdots are marked on the cut surface of the vas deferens and two parallel double-armed sutures are placed in the distended epididymal tubule longitudinally and parallel to each other (Fig. 9.1a, b); however, **the needles are not pulled through. If they are pulled through prior to placing the second needle and making the opening in the epididymal tubule, sperm will leak from the needle hole** because the needle is 70 μm in diameter, and the suture is only 17 μm in diameter. This will cause the epididymal tubule to collapse, making placement of the second needle and incising the tubule more difficult. After the epididymal fluid is tested for sperm, if motile, it is aspirated into micropipettes for cryopreservation. The two needles in the epididymal tubule are then pulled through, and all four needles are placed through the vasal lumen exiting through the 4 microdots (Fig. 9.2). Prior to tying the 10-0 sutures, a stay suture is placed with 9-0 nylon to bring the vasal lumen down directly above the opening in the epididymal tubule, taking all tension off before tying (Fig. 9.3). **Prior to tying the 10-0 sutures, the surgeon must see the free end move**, thereby assuring there are no loops and no slack just prior to tying. This assures that the epididymal tubule wall is plastered against the vasal mucosa and is intussuscepted into the vasal lumen. After the 10-0 sutures are tied, eight to twelve 9-0 nylon sutures are placed from the edge of the opening in the epididymal tunic to the vasal muscularis and adventitia (Fig. 9.4). The patency rate with the LIVE approach has been reported at 66.1–90% and is the preferred method for all vasoepididymostomies [2, 6, 7].

Tips

All successful vasovasostomy and vasoepididymostomy techniques rely on adherence to surgical principles that are universally applicable to anastomoses of all tubular structures:

1. Accurate approximation of healthy mucosa-to-mucosa, yielding a leak-proof anastomosis.
2. Tension-free anastomosis; good blood supply to the vas and epididymis and muscularis.

M. Goldstein, *Atlas of Male Infertility Microsurgery*, https://doi.org/10.1007/978-3-031-31601-2_9

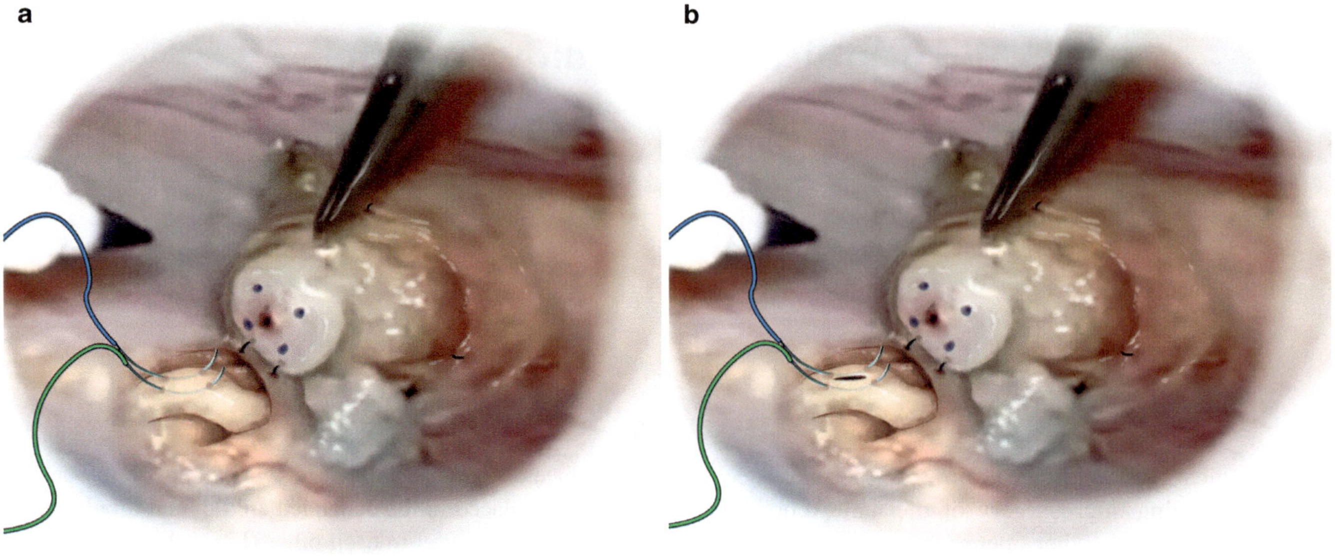

Fig. 9.1 (**a**, **b**) Four microdots are marked on the cut surface of the vas deferens and two parallel double-armed sutures are placed in the distended epididymal tubule longitudinally and parallel to each other

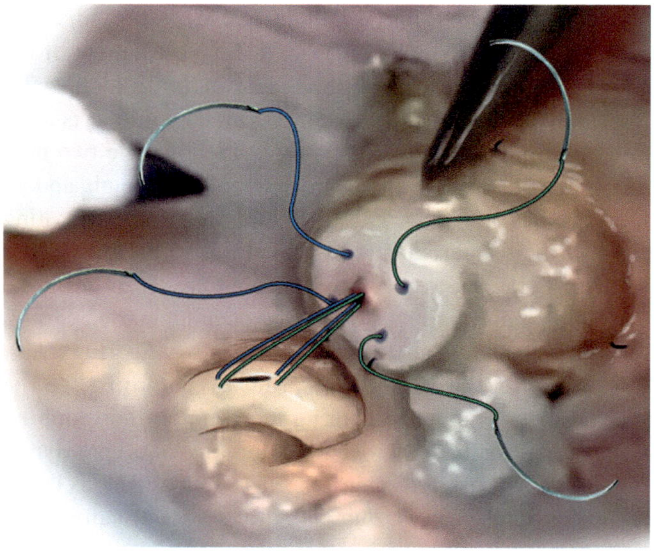

Fig. 9.2 Two needles in the epididymal tubule are pulled through, and all four needles are placed through the vasal lumen exiting through the four microdots

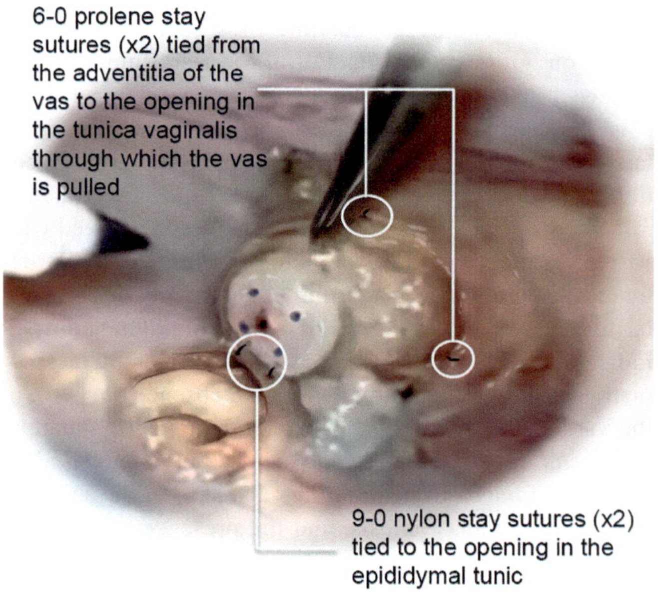

Fig. 9.3 Before tying the 10-0 sutures, a stay suture is placed with 9-0 nylon to bring the vasal lumen down directly above the opening in the epididymal tubule, taking all tension off before tying

3. The same tips for vasovasostomy apply to vasoepididymostomy.
4. The 9-0 stay suture bringing the vas right over the epididymal tubule is critical before tying. Tying mycosal sutures without that stay suture will likely cause the epididymal suture to tear out when tying.
5. Before tying the 10-0 mucosal sutures, you must see the free end move. This ensures there is no slack and that the epididymal mucosa is plastered against the wall of the vasal mucosa before tying.

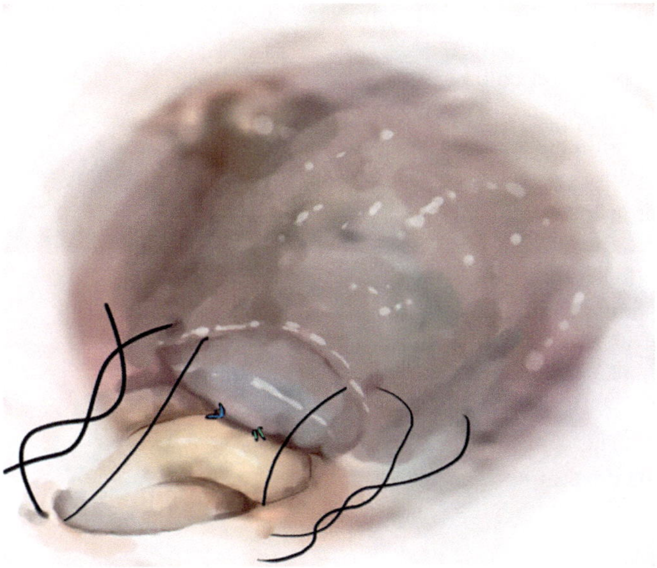

Fig. 9.4 After the 10-0 sutures are tied, eight to twelve 9-0 nylon sutures are placed from the edge of the opening in the epididymal tunic to the vasal muscularis and adventitia

References

1. Goldstein M. Surgical management of male infertility. In: Wein AJ, et al., editors. Campbell-Walsh urology. Philadelphia, PA: Elsevier; 2016. p. 580–611.
2. Hong K, et al. Multiple factors affecting surgical outcomes and patency rates in use of single-armed two-suture microsurgical vasoepididymostomy: a single surgeon's experience with 81 patients. Asian J Androl. 2016;18:129–33.
3. Berger R. Triangulation end-to-side vasoepididymostomy. J Urol. 1998;159(6):1951–3.
4. Marmar J. Modified vasoepididymostomy with simultaneous double needle placement, tubulotomy and tubular invagination. J Urol. 2000;163(2):483–6.
5. Chan PTK, Li PS, Goldstein M. Microsurgical vasoepididymostomy: a prospective randomized study of three intussusception techniques in rats. J Urol. 2003;169:1924–9.
6. Peng J, et al. Pregnancy and live birth rates after microsurgical vasoepididymostomy for azoospermic patients with epididymal obstruction. Hum Reprod. 2017;32(2):284–9.
7. Chan PTK, Brandell R, Goldstein M. Prospective analysis of outcomes after microsurgical intussusception vaso-epididymostomy. BJUI Int. 2005;96:598–601.

10 Microsurgical Epididymal Sperm Aspiration

Two major discoveries in the treatment of male infertility have allowed the treatment of men with a surgically unreconstructable reproductive tract obstruction. The first of these is the introduction of intracytoplasmic sperm injection. The second discovery is the finding that sperm retrieval either from the epididymis or from the testicle can yield sperm which are usable with a good possibility for pregnancy and live births utilizing IVF/ICSI. Candidates for microsurgical epididymal sperm aspiration (MESA) are men with congenital or acquired reproductive tract obstruction. Unrepairable obstructions include men with congenital bilateral absence of the vas deferens, microsurgically unreconstructable reproductive tract obstruction or men who choose to have primary treatment with microsurgical epididymal sperm retrieval, rather than reproductive tract reconstruction. It provides several benefits over percutaneous sperm retrieval techniques. First, certainty of sperm retrieval with MESA is over 99% of cases. It provides the opportunity to have millions of viable sperm cryopreserved in multiple vials for subsequent attempts at fertility using IVF/ICSI. Finally, it allows retrieval of sperm from multiple sources (e.g., right and left epididymis and right and left testis, and possibly even vasal sperm) with DNA integrity testing performed on samples from each source (we use the TUNEL assay), allowing us to tell the IVF doctor which samples to use for IVF/ICSI providing the highest possibility of live birth.

In patients who have had multiple failed IVF cycles, and the sperm DNA integrity of semen is very poor, surgical retrieval of sperm from the testicle and possibly from the efferent ducts, invariably results in better sperm DNA integrity than the ejaculated sperm. These specimens can then be used for IVF/ICSI.

10.1 Procedure

The surgeon's non-dominant hand gently grasps the testis while stabilizing the epididymis between thumb and index finger. Using the operating microscope at 10–15× magnification, the microtipped bipolar forceps are used to create an avascular spot in the epididymal tunic overlying dilated, golden-clear fluid containing tubules, usually in the caput. Tubules appearing to be filled with thick, yellow material usually contain only sperm heads and debris and should be avoided. A 3.5 mm buttonhole opening is made in the tunic by elevating it with a jeweler's forceps and excising a wedge of the epididymal tunic with micro-scissors, taking care to keep the underlying epididymal tubules intact (Fig. 10.1). Hemostasis is attained using the microbipolar forceps. A dilated epididymal tubule is selected and isolated with gentle dissection using a microneedle holder (Fig. 10.2). The tubule is then punctured with a 15° microknife (Fig. 10.3). The epididymal fluid is touched to a sterile glass slide (Fig. 10.4), a

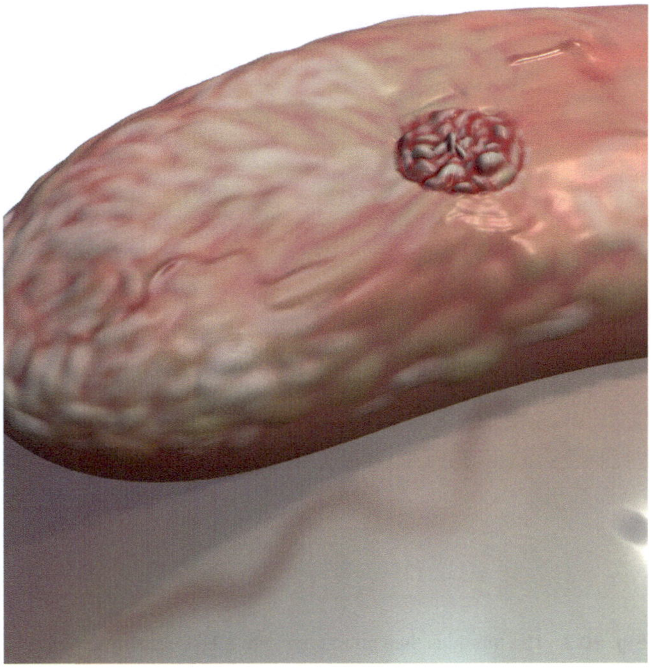

Fig. 10.1 A 3.5 mm buttonhole opening is made in the tunic by elevating it with a jeweler's forceps and excising a wedge of the epididymal tunic with micro-scissors, taking care to keep the underlying epididymal tubules intact

M. Goldstein, *Atlas of Male Infertility Microsurgery*, https://doi.org/10.1007/978-3-031-31601-2_10

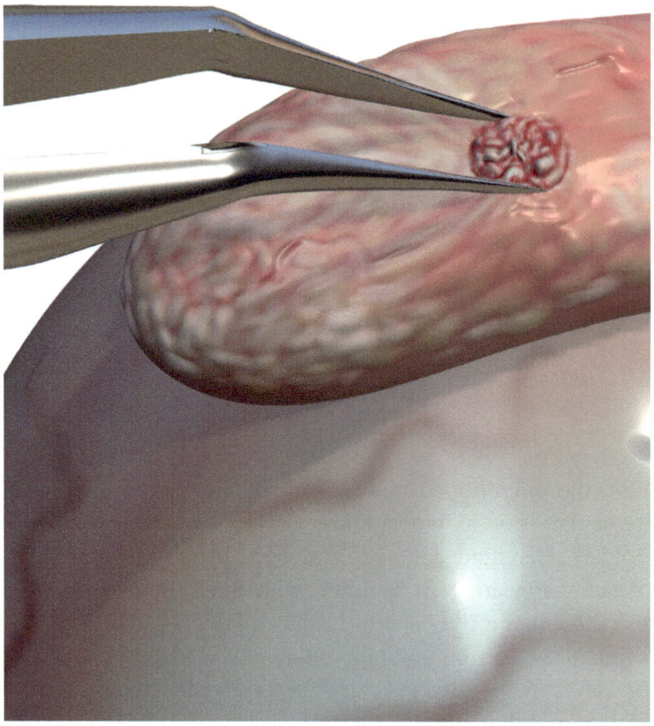

Fig. 10.2 A dilated epididymal tubule is selected and isolated with gentle dissection using a microneedle holder

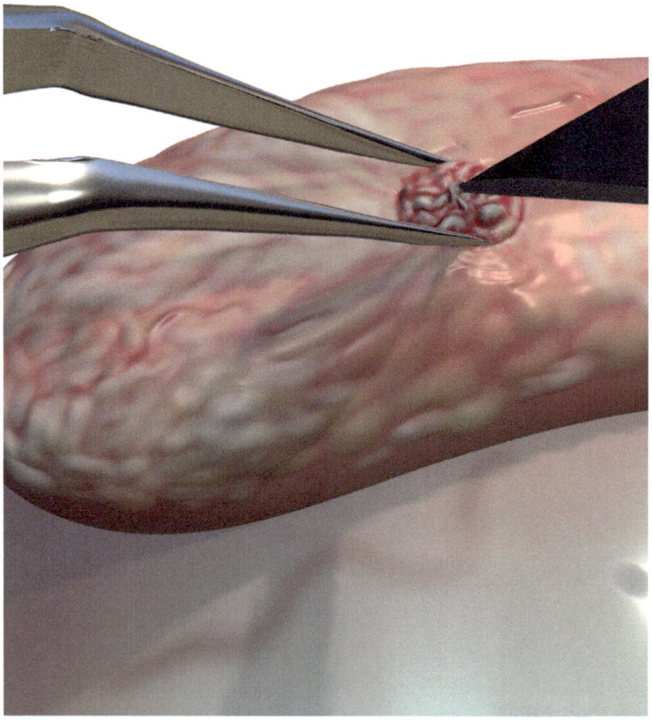

Fig. 10.3 The tubule is then punctured with a 15-degree microknife

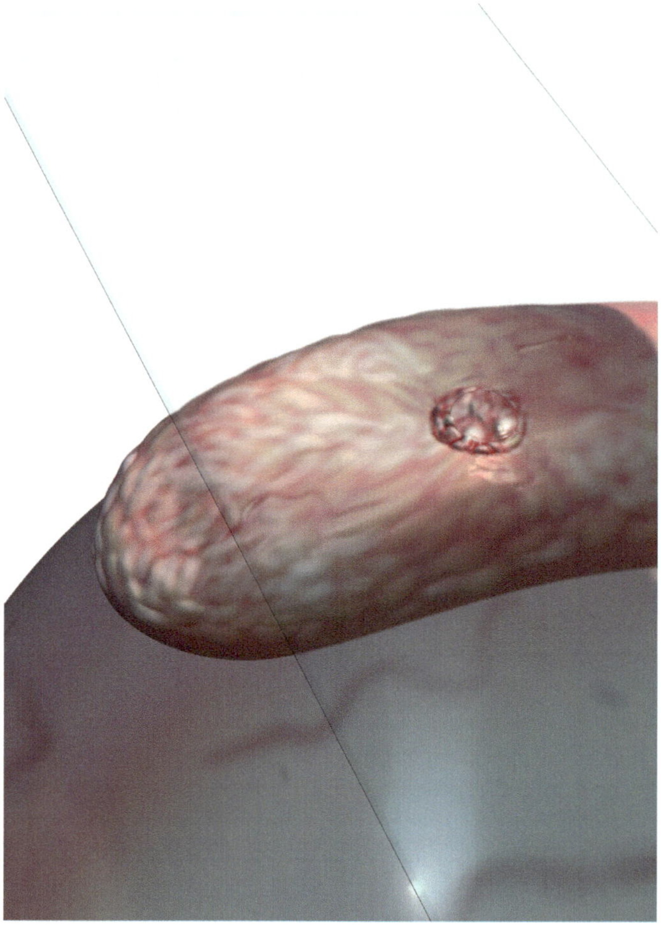

Fig. 10.4 The epididymal fluid is touched to a sterile glass slide, a drop of human tubal fluid is added and a cover slip is placed over the fluid, then the sample is immediately examined under the separate 400 power bench microscope

drop of human tubal fluid is added and a cover slip is placed over the fluid, then the sample is immediately examined under the separate 400 power bench microscope. In an obstructed epididymis, sperm within the more caudal aspect of the epididymis tend to be of poorer quality. Better quality sperm are usually found within the caput. Puncture of multiple tubules may be necessary to find the best quality sperm. When motile sperm are identified, a dry micropipette (5 μL; Drummond Scientific Co., Broomall, PA) or standard hematocrit pipette is placed adjacent to the effluxing epididymal tubule to capture the sperm-containing fluid (Fig. 10.5). The epididymal fluid will be drawn into the pipette by simple capillary action.

The highest rate of flow from the epididymis is observed immediately after incising the tubule. Sperm quality progressively improves after initial washout. Gentle compression of

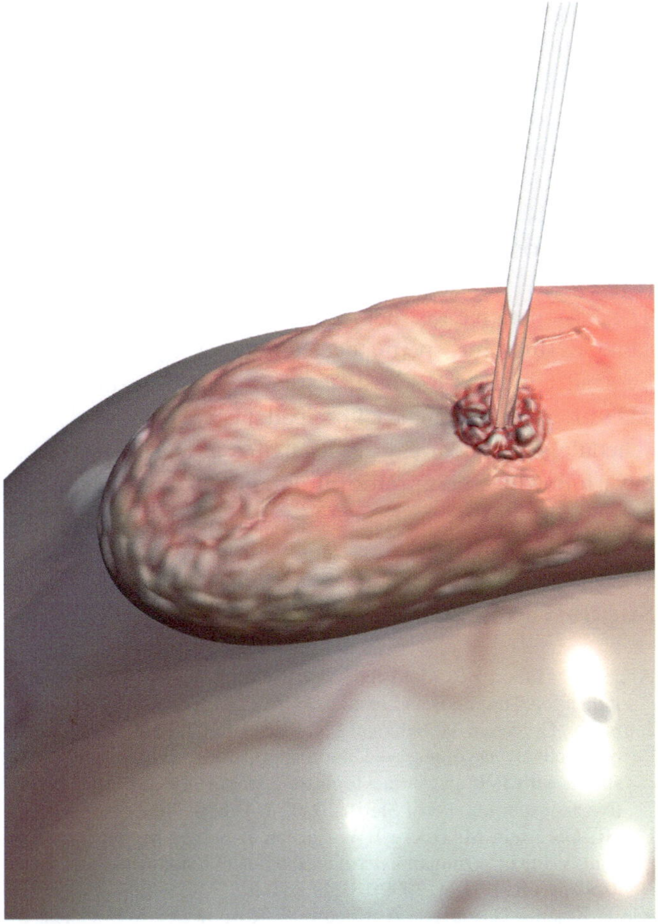

Fig. 10.5 A dry micropipette or standard hematocrit pipette is placed adjacent to the effluxing epididymal tubule to capture the sperm-containing fluid

the epididymis and testis using the stabilizing thumb and index finger can enhance flow from the tubule. With patience, 25–50 μL of highly concentrated epididymal fluid can be recovered, containing a total of approximately 75 million sperm divided into 6–15 vials for cryopreservation. If no sperm or only immotile sperm are obtained at the initial incision site or if the quantities of sperm acquired are inadequate, additional incisions are made more proximally along the epididymis or even at the level of the efferent ductules until motile sperm are obtained. The extracted fluid is diluted in multiple aliquots of 0.5–1 mL of human tubal fluid (HTF) medium. One specimen from each site undergoes post-freeze/thaw motility assessment, and TUNEL assay.

Once sufficient quantities of good quality sperm are obtained, the tubular incisions are sealed using bipolar cautery and meticulous hemostasis is attained. The testis and epididymis are returned to the tunica vaginalis, which is closed with a running 5-0 Vicryl suture. The testis is reduced into the hemi-scrotum and the scrotal incision is closed in layers with a subcuticular skin closure. Bacitracin ointment is placed on the wound and fluffed gauze is held in place with an athletic supporter.

10.2 Complications

Complications after epididymal aspiration procedure are very rare. They include wound infection, scrotal hematoma, epididymal scarring, and injury to the epididymal and spermatic cord vasculature which might possibly lead to testis atrophy and/or impaired testis function. Scrotal exploration is rarely indicated for management of any of these complications. Given the blind nature of percutaneous epididymal sperm aspiration (PESA), risks of scrotal hematoma, scarring, and vessel injury are higher than those associated with MESA.

Tips

- Unreconstructable azoospermia, once untreatable, with patients relegated to donor sperm or adoption, are now the diagnosis with the highest live birth rates of all etiologies of male factor infertility. This is primary in vitro *fertilization* (IVF) with intracytoplasmic sperm injection (ICSI) combined with advanced techniques of microsurgical sperm aspiration.
- If one is unable to palpate either vas deferens on physical examination, the cause of obstruction is CBAVD.
- Screening for the CFTR gene mutation should be performed both in the patient and his partner and genetic counseling provided as needed.
- In patients with suspected or known obstructive azoospermia who exhibit testicular atrophy on exam and/or elevated FSH with serum testing, testis biopsy may be considered to confirm normal spermatogenesis.
- Men with suspected obstructive azoospermia and palpable vasa should have serum antisperm antibody testing which, if highly positive, has a high predictive accuracy of azoospermia secondary to obstruction and obviates the need for a testis biopsy.
- Tubules appearing to be filled with thick, yellow material usually contains only sperm heads and debris and should be avoided.
- When motile sperm are identified, a dry micropipette (5 μL; Drummond Scientific Co., Broomall, PA) or standard hematocrit pipette is placed adjacent to the effluxing epididymal tubule to capture the sperm-containing fluid. The epididymal fluid will be drawn into the pipette by simple capillary action.
- Percutaneous epididymal sperm aspiration (PESA) has variable success rates for sperm retrieval, averaging 80%,

and does not generally yield numbers of sperm sufficient to allow for cryopreservation and, for that reason, should be performed contemporaneously with egg retrieval.

- Gentle compression of the epididymis and testis using the stabilizing thumb and index finger can enhance flow from the tubule.
- The ability to cryopreserve sperm obtained from men with obstructive azoospermia can help allay concerns regarding coordination of sperm extraction with timing of oocyte retrieval and also offers the possibility of avoidance of repeat sperm retrieval procedures if good quantities of motile sperm are obtained at the initial extraction. The higher yields of sperm associated with MESA as compared with PESA allow cryopreservation of multiple vials of sperm sufficient for multiple IVF-ICSI cycles.

10.3 Conclusion

The ability to cryopreserve sperm obtained from men with obstructive azoospermia can help allay concerns regarding coordination of sperm extraction with timing of oocyte retrieval and also minimizes the need for repeat sperm retrieval procedures if good quantities of motile sperm are obtained at the initial extraction. The higher yields of sperm associated with MESA as compared with percutaneous retrieval allow cryopreservation of multiple vials of sperm sufficient for multiple IVF-ICSI cycles. No differences in outcomes comparing use of fresh or cryopreserved/thawed sperm have been observed.

In the hands of an experienced microsurgeon, MESA offers 99% sperm retrieval rates and 70% live delivery rates in conjunction with IVF/ICSI. In addition, cryopreservation of retrieved sperm adds further convenience and flexibility in terms of cycle planning.

10.4 Postoperative Instructions

The postoperative instructions for sperm aspiration are the same as that for spermatocelectomy or hydrocelectomy. Typically, it takes ten business days for the results of the TUNEL assay to come back, so patients are instructed to not schedule subsequent egg retrievals for at least ten business days following sperm retrieval unless they are planning on cryopreserving oocytes.

Suggested Reading

Anger JT, Gilbert BR, Goldstein MARC. Cryopreservation of sperm: indications, methods and results. J Urol. 2003;170(4):1079–84.

Janzen N, Goldstein M, Schlegel PN, Palermo GD, Rosenwaks Z. Use of electively cryopreserved microsurgically aspirated epididymal sperm with IVF and intracytoplasmic sperm injection for obstructive azoospermia. Fertil Steril. 2000;74(4):696–701.

Lee R, Goldstein M, Ullery BW, Ehrlich J, Soares M, Razzano RA, et al. Value of serum antisperm antibodies in diagnosing obstructive azoospermia. J Urol. 2009;181(1):264–9.

Xie P, Keating D, Parrella A, Cheung S, Rosenwaks Z, Goldstein M, Palermo GD. Sperm genomic integrity by TUNEL varies throughout the male genital tract. J Urol. 2020;203(4):802–8.

11 Microsurgical Testicular Sperm Retrieval

Diagnostic testis biopsy to distinguish obstructive from non-obstructive azoospermia (NOA) is rarely indicated. Testis biopsy is more often performed to retrieve testicular sperm for IVF/ICSI. Using an operating microscope minimizes the risk of bleeding or accidental injury to the epididymis or testicular blood supply. Microsurgical testis biopsy is less painful, and more likely to obtain good tissue while being much less likely to injure the testicular blood supply or epididymis than blind percutaneous testicular biopsy. Microdissection TESE sperm retrieval in non-obstructive azoospermia has made possible oocyte fertilization with even minimal numbers of sperm with limited intrinsic fertilizing capacity. After completing his fellowship with me and joining our department, I convinced Dr. Peter Schlegel to employ an operating microscope when doing a testis biopsy, primarily to identify and avoid injury to the sub-tunical testicular blood supply [1, 2]. This led to his development of the groundbreaking technique of microTESE for non-obstructive azoospermia. His video describing this technique is available on the Weill Cornell Brady Urology YouTube channel.

11.1 Procedure

Microsurgical testicular sperm retrieval for patients with obstructive azoospermia begins with an initial incision and exposure of the testis identical to that for microsurgical epididymal sperm retrieval. Once the testis is delivered, a 7 mm incision site in the tunica albuginea between sub-tunical vessels is cauterized with the micro-bipolar cautery. Using a 15° microknife, incise the tunica albuginea in the bipolared area until seminiferous tubules extrude (Fig. 11.1). Excise the tissue with a curved iris scissor, the curve of the scissors matching the curve of the testis so that maximum amount of tissue is excised (Fig. 11.2). The micro-bipolar electrocautery is used to control bleeders. Reapproximate the tunica albuginea with two or three interrupted sutures of 5-0 Vicryl. Return the testis to the tunica vaginalis and close in the usual fashion.

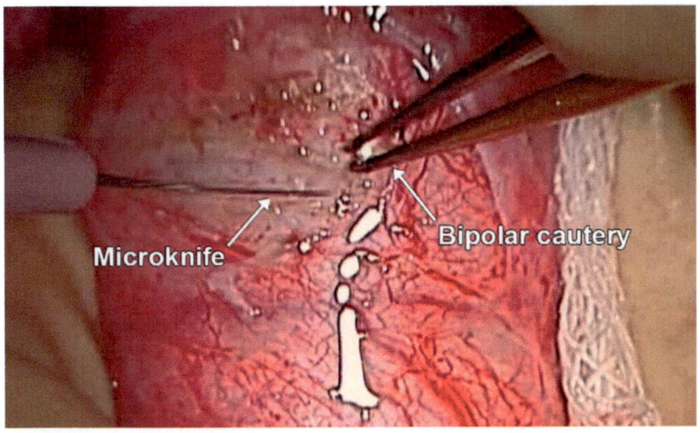

Fig. 11.1 Using a 15° microknife, incise the tunica albuginea in the bipolared area until seminiferous tubules extrude

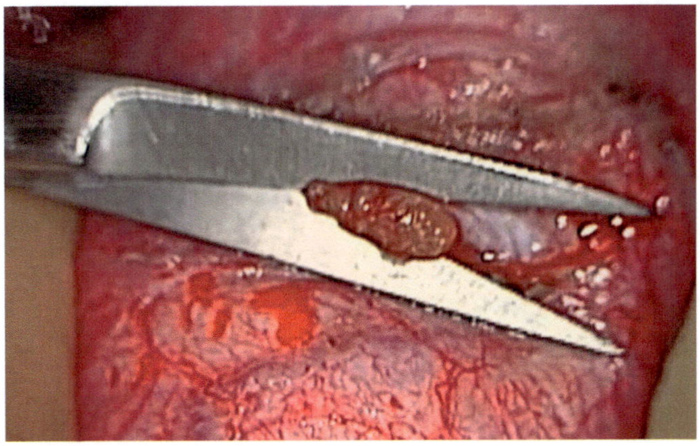

Fig. 11.2 Excise the tissue with a curved iris scissor, the curve of the scissors matching the curve of the testis so that maximum amount of tissue is excised

Tips

1. Use interrupted sutures to reapproximate the incision in the tunica albuginea. This way if there is bleeding, it is better for it to come out, rather than cause intratesticular hematoma.

M. Goldstein, *Atlas of Male Infertility Microsurgery*, https://doi.org/10.1007/978-3-031-31601-2_11

2. When doing a diagnostic biopsy, always regard it as a potential therapeutic biopsy (i.e., always cryopreserve tissue for possible use for IVF/ICSI).
3. Use the fewest stitches possible: two, or at the most three sutures to close the tunica albuginea incision. The unnecessary extra suture is always the one that goes through a blood vessel and bleeds.

References

1. Schlegel P, et al. Testicular sperm extraction with ICSI for non-obstructive azoospermia. Urology. 1997;49:435–40.
2. Dardashti K, Williams RH, Goldstein M. Microsurgical testis biopsy: a novel technique for retrieval of testicular tissue. J Urol. 2000;163(4):1206–7.

12 Transurethral Resection of the Ejaculatory Ducts (TURED)

Obstruction of the ejaculatory ducts accounts for approximately 5% of obstructive azoospermia cases. Ejaculatory duct obstruction is suspected in men with obstructive azoospermia with at least one palpable vas deferens, a low semen volume, acidic semen pH and negative, equivocal, or low semen fructose levels. Transrectal ultrasound should be performed immediately before anticipated surgery. Midline cysts and dilatation of the seminal vesicles can be visualized. The dilated seminal vesicles are aspirated under ultrasound guidance and the fluid is examined under the microscope. Motile sperm can be cryopreserved for later use. Indigo carmine diluted with water-soluble radiographic contrast material is instilled. If a potentially resectable lesion is confirmed, transurethral resection of the ejaculatory ducts can be performed without prior vasography. However, if no sperm are found in the aspirate, a vasogram must be performed. A vasogram (see Chap. 7) should only be performed by urologists with microsurgical experience, who can proceed with reconstruction at the same time.

The left and right ejaculatory ducts enter the prostatic urethra at the level of the utricle. TURED should not be considered a benign procedure, as it is occasionally associated with significant morbidity, most commonly contamination of semen with urine. Normally, ejaculatory ducts contain a valve-like mechanism that prevents reflux of urine into the ejaculatory duct. After TURED, a significant percentage of men will develop reflux of urine up the excurrent ductal system, causing chemical and/or bacterial epididymitis.

A successful TURED must first begin with a vasotomy and vasogram for precise identification of the ejaculatory ducts. See Chap. 7 for a description of vasography technique.

12.1 Procedure

The vas deferens is isolated at the junction of the straight and convoluted portions. Under ten power magnification, a clean segment of vas is surrounded with a vessel loop and a straight clamp is placed beneath the vas to act as a platform (see Chap. 7). Under 25 power magnification, a 15-degree microknife is used to hemi-transect the vas (Fig. 7.1a). Fluid exuding from the lumen is placed on a slide for microscopic examination using a separate bench microscope under 400× magnification. The presence of sperm or sperm parts confirms absence of epididymal obstruction. If motile sperm are found, they are aspirated and cryopreserved. The end of the vas toward the seminal vesicles is cannulated with a 24-gauge angio-catheter sheath and is injected with 1 mL of lactated ringers' solution to test its patency (Fig. 7.2). Next, 1 mL of 50% dilute indigo carmine is injected with a number 16 French Foley catheter in the bladder. The absence of dye in the urine confirms obstruction of the outflow tract. Vasography is performed by passing a number 3 whistle-tip ureteral catheter toward the seminal vesicle end of the vas and 0.5 mL of water-soluble contrast media is injected. This patient's vasogram revealed markedly dilated seminal vesicles and a midline ejaculatory duct cyst, findings for ejaculatory duct obstruction ideal for potential TURED (see Fig. 7.5). If ejaculatory duct obstruction is confirmed by vasography, the number three French whistle tip ureteral stents are left in place so that dilute indigo carmine solution can be injected by the assistant to aid resection. The resectoscope with a 24 French cutting loop is engaged with a finger placed in the rectum providing anterior displacement of the posterior lobe of the prostate. The ejaculatory ducts exit along the lateral aspect of the verumontanum (Fig. 12.1). Resection of the verumontanum will often reveal the dilated ejaculatory duct orifice or cyst cavity. Resection should be carried out with great care to preserve the bladder neck proximally, the external sphincter distally and the rectal mucosa posteriorly (Fig. 12.2). Efflux of indigo carmine from dilated orifices confirms adequate resection, excessive coagulation should be avoided. The hemi-transected vasography sites are carefully closed microsurgically using two or three interrupted sutures of 10-0 monofilament nylon for the mucosa, and 9-0 for the muscularis and adventitia. A Foley catheter is left in overnight, and the patient receives an additional 7 days of oral antibiotic therapy.

M. Goldstein, *Atlas of Male Infertility Microsurgery*, https://doi.org/10.1007/978-3-031-31601-2_12

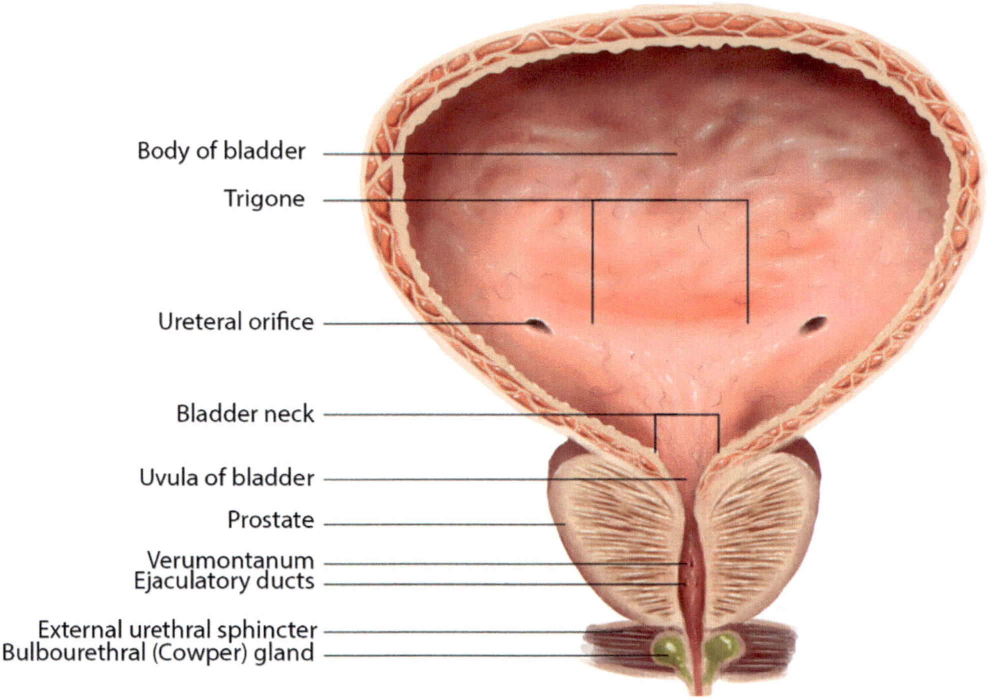

Fig. 12.1 The ejaculatory ducts exit along the lateral aspect of the verumontanum

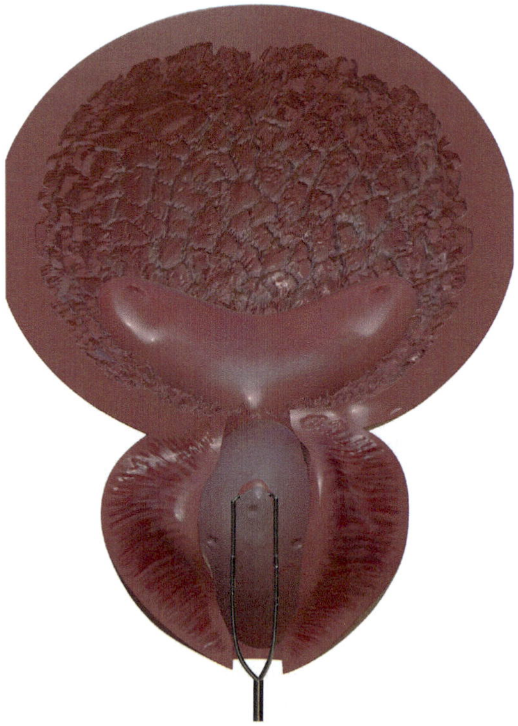

Fig. 12.2 Resection should be carried out with great care to preserve the bladder neck proximally, the external sphincter distally and the rectal mucosa posteriorly

12.2 Complications

Reflux of urine into the reproductive tract is common after this procedure. This can be confirmed by measuring semen creatinine. Urine reflux can have detrimental effects on sperm quality reflux of urine can also lead to epididymitis both acute and chronic. Retrograde ejaculation is another common complication of transurethral resection. Pseudoephedrine 120 mg orally 90 min before ejaculation may reverse retrograde ejaculation. Because of the potential for serious complications, transurethral resection should be performed only on carefully selected well-informed patients, who would prefer this procedure to IVF/ICSI with surgically retrieved sperm.

12.3 Conclusion

Although not a common diagnosis, obstruction of the ejaculatory ducts is a potentially surgically treatable cause of obstructive azoospermia. Careful patient selection and surgical preparation are important for successful treatment.

Suggested Reading

Vazquez-Levin MH, Dressler KP, Nagler HM. Urine contamination of seminal fluid after transurethral resection of the ejaculatory ducts. J Urol. 1994;152(6):2049–52.

13 Testis-Sparing Excision of Testicular Tumor

Radical orchiectomy is indicated for palpable testis tumors because of a majority of these are malignant. Impalpable testis tumors found incidentally on ultrasound are found to be benign in over 50% of cases [1]. In men with a solitary testis or a contralateral atrophic or poorly functioning testis, radical orchiectomy will render such men sterile and, often, androgen deficient. We developed a technique of ultrasound, needle-guided microsurgical enucleation of such tumors allowing preservation of the testis. Even when the tumor turns out to be malignant, no men have developed metastasis or have had recurrence requiring later radical orchiectomy [2].

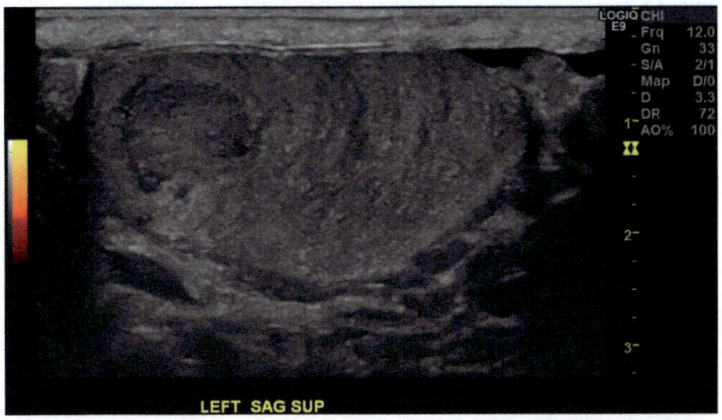

Fig. 13.1 The intratesticular mass is localized with sonography

13.1 Procedure

The testis is delivered through an inguinal incision. The gubernaculum is clamped. Ice saline slush solution is placed around the testis for 10 min before a rubber-shod vascular clamp is placed across the spermatic cord to minimize warm ischemia. The tunica vaginalis is opened and the testicle is exposed. The testicle remains on ice throughout the duration of the procedure. The gubernacular vessels are occluded with a hemostat. The intratesticular mass is localized with sonography using a Sequoia 512 unit (Acuson, Mountain View, California) and linear transducer at 15 MHz (Fig. 13.1). Under real-time ultrasound, a 30-gauge needle is placed adjacent to the lesion. Small blood vessels subjacent to the tunica albuginea are identified with the operating microscope, providing 6–25× magnification. A 15-degee ultra sharp microknife is used to make an incision within a relatively avascular region of the tunica. Seminiferous tubules adjacent to the needle are separated carefully by blunt dissection with a micro-needle holder until the mass is visualized. The lesion is excised, leaving a 2–5 mm shell of normal appearing testicular parenchyma around the mass. Benign tumors typically pop out easily like a small grape (Fig. 13.2). Malignant ones are usually more adhered to the surrounding tissue. The lesion is sent for frozen tissue analysis.

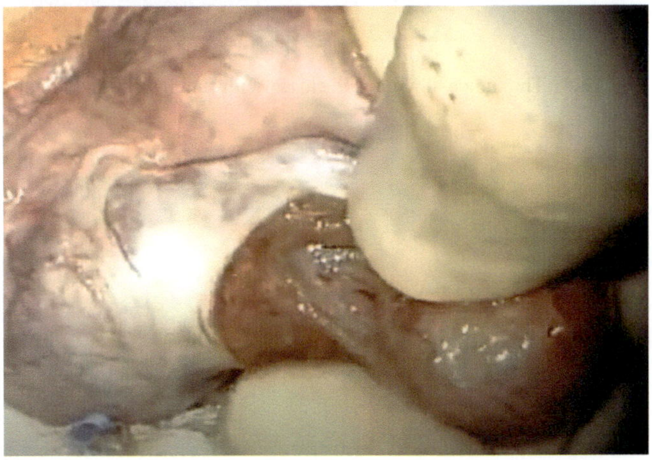

Fig. 13.2 Benign tumors typically pop out easily like a small grape

If pathological findings are benign, the vascular clamp on the spermatic cord and hemostat across the gubernaculum are removed. The parenchyma and tunica are inspected for hemostasis, which may be achieved with bipolar electrocautery (Fig. 13.3). If pathological findings are malignant, radical orchiectomy may be done, while in cases of bilateral malignancy or a neoplasm within a solitary testis, the testis preserving approach may be used. Multiple biopsies of the

M. Goldstein, *Atlas of Male Infertility Microsurgery*, https://doi.org/10.1007/978-3-031-31601-2_13

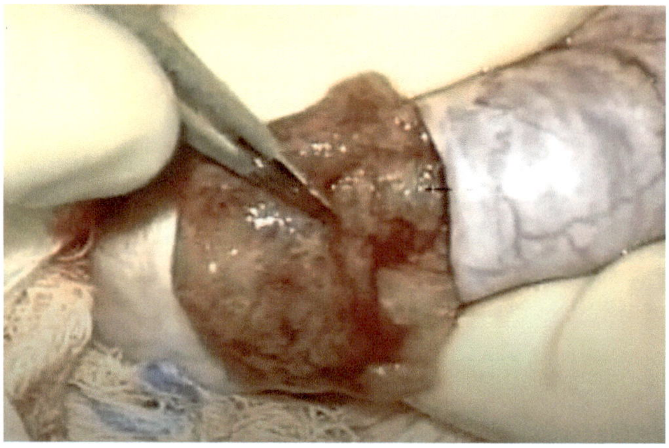

Fig. 13.3 Hemostasis is achieved with bipolar electrocautery

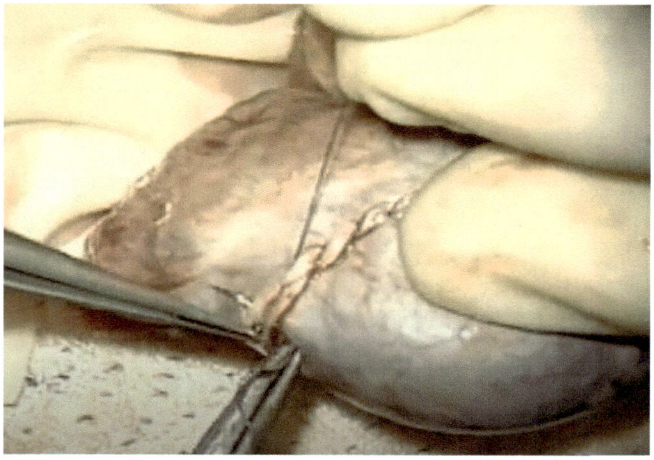

Fig. 13.4 The tunica albuginea is closed with running 5-0 polyglactin suture

remaining parenchyma are done to ensure absent malignancy and assess intratubular germ cell neoplasia on permanent section.

The testis and wound are irrigated with sterile water to lyse any potentially malignant spilled cells. The tunica albuginea is closed with running 5-0 polyglactin suture (Fig. 13.4). Negative margins of the specimen containing the tumor are confirmed by permanent tissue analysis.

13.2 Complications

Prophylactic antibiotics (2 g Ancef IV) prior to incision suffices to prevent infection. Meticulous hemostasis with the bipolar cautery and careful closure of the biopsy site prevents intratesticular hematoma.

References

1. Eifler J, King P, Schlegel P. Incidental testicular lesions found during infertility evaluation are usually benign and may be managed conservatively. J Urol. 2008;180:261–5.
2. Hopps C, Goldstein M. Ultrasound guided needle localization and microsurgical exploration for incidental nonpalpable testicular tumors. J Urol. 2002;168:1084–7.

14 Microsurgically Assisted Repair of Inguinal Hernia

Inguinal hernia repairs are the most performed general surgery procedures with 800,000 performed per year in the United States and 20 million worldwide. Furthermore, hernia repairs are the most common cause of iatrogenic obstruction of the vas deferens and impaired testicular blood supply. Chronic inguinal pain more than 3 months post-op is common and very difficult to treat. It is thought to be due to intraoperative nerve entrapment, stretching, or thermal injury. Our rationale for using an operating microscope to assist inguinal hernia repair is to provide significantly improved visualization of anatomical structures therefore avoiding injury to the ilioinguinal nerve, genital branch of the genitofemoral nerve, vas deferens and its nerves, or testicular blood supply and to allow for more precise control of small vessels and hemostasis with a bipolar micro-cautery [1].

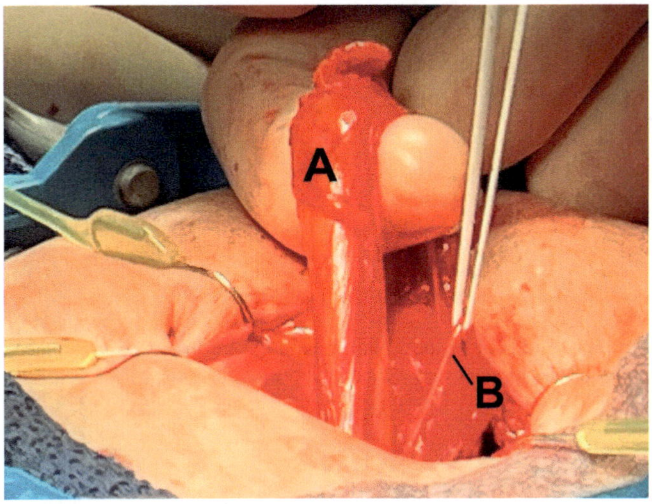

Fig. 14.1 The spermatic cord (**a**) exiting the external ring, prior to opening the ring, with the ilioinguinal nerve (**b**) isolated with a white vessel loop

14.1 Procedure

A 4.5 cm inguinal incision is made within Langer's lines (see Fig. 2.1). Gentamicin solution is sprayed into the wound at skin opening and throughout the case. Campers and Scarpa's fascia are divided with a Bovie electrocautery. The superficial epigastric artery and vein are divided and ligated with 3-0 Vicryl. The external oblique aponeurosis is exposed with sweeping blunt dissection. A self-retaining Scott retractor is introduced to maintain exposure. The operating microscope is brought into the field. Under 6–25 power magnification, the ilioinguinal nerve is identified exiting the external inguinal ring (Fig. 14.1) and a vessel loop is placed around it for identification. The spermatic cord is isolated and the vas deferens is visualized and palpated throughout the case to avoid injury to it or its blood supply. A Penrose drain is then placed around the cord, which is explored anterio-medially for an indirect sac or large lipoma. An indirect hernia sac found within the external spermatic fascia is identified by a white colored edge (Fig. 14.2a). An example of a direct hernia sac is shown in Fig. 14.2b. The sac is dissected off of the cord under ten power magnification with the combination of blunt and sharp dissection to the internal ring. It usually is found adjacent to, and stuck to, the vas deferens. After opening it and reducing its contents, the sac is doubly ligated with 2-0 silk and excised. It will retract into the retroperitoneum. The internal ring is then tightened with interrupted to 2-0 absorbable monofilament sutures to a diameter that can accommodate the cord and a pinky finger (Fig. 14.3). For a direct hernia, the contents are reduced, and the defect is plugged with a Betadine-soaked polyethylene plug which may be secured with an absorbable suture if the defect is large (Fig. 14.4). A polyethylene patch is soaked in Betadine and placed on the floor of the inguinal canal with a 1.25 cm diameter pre-cut round opening for the spermatic cord to pass through (Fig. 14.5). The proximal leaves of the mesh are secured loosely to each other over the cord. Care is taken to ensure the mesh lies flat with no folds; 2-0 absorbable monofilament sutures is used to secure the mesh to the pubic tubercle inferiorly with an interrupted mattress

M. Goldstein, *Atlas of Male Infertility Microsurgery*, https://doi.org/10.1007/978-3-031-31601-2_14

Fig. 14.2 (**a**) An indirect hernia sac found within the external spermatic fascia is identified by a white colored edge. (**b**) An example of a direct hernia sac. (**c**) Intraoperative image of a direct hernia sac

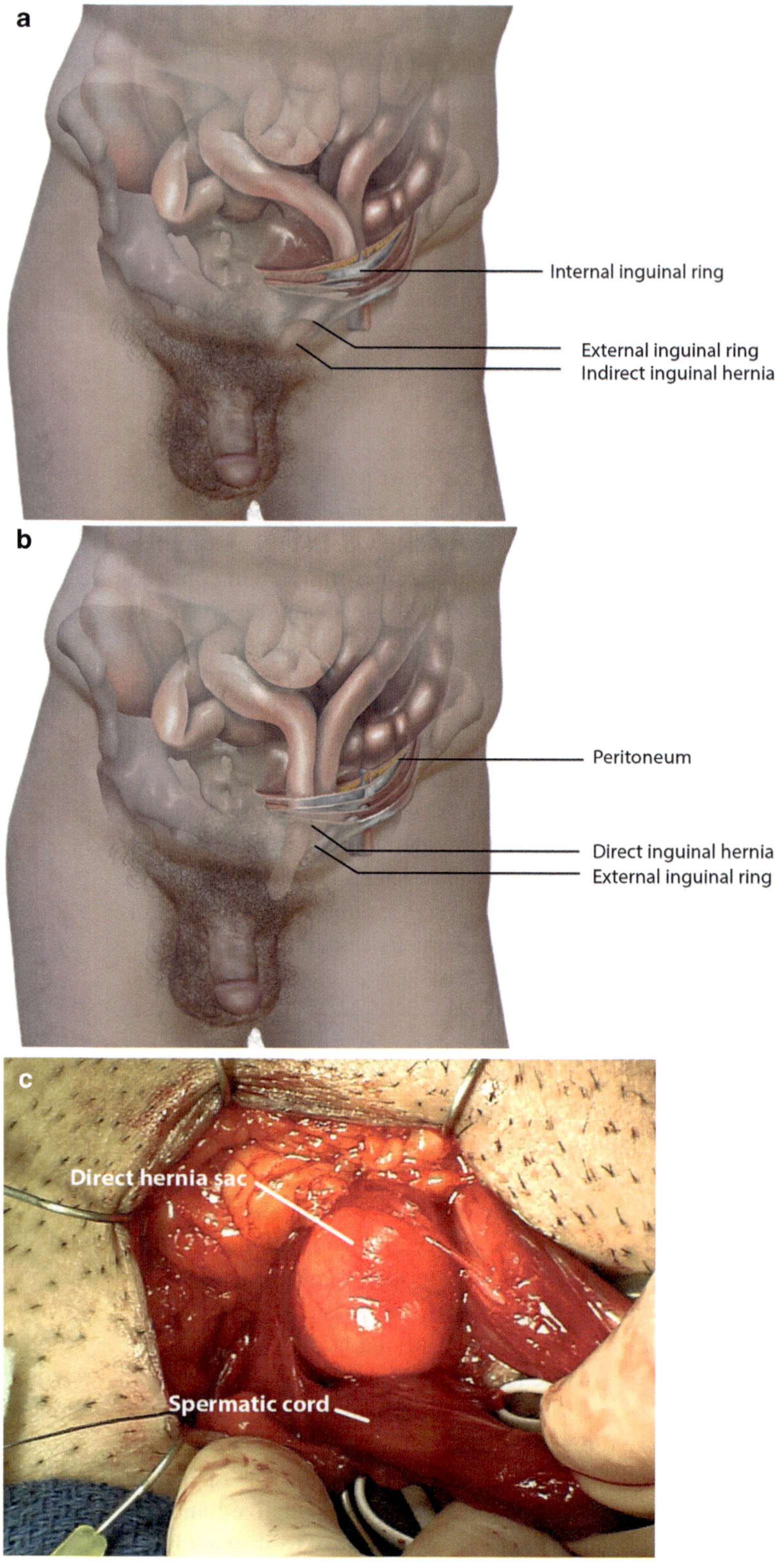

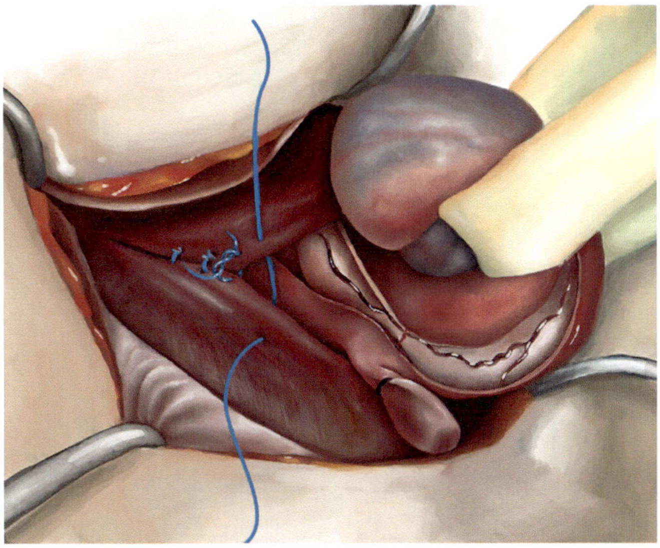

Fig. 14.3 The internal ring is then tightened with an interrupted 2-0 absorbable monofilament suture to a diameter that can accommodate the cord and your pinky finger. (From Schulster et al. [1]; with permission)

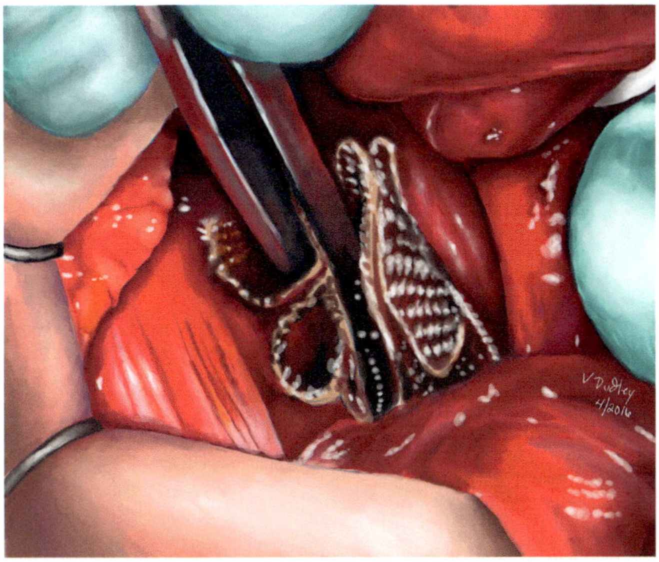

Fig. 14.4 The defect is plugged with a Betadine-soaked polyethylene plug which may be secured with an absorbable suture if the defect is large. (From Schulster et al. [1]; with permission)

suture. The cord is returned to its bed over the mesh and the opening is inspected to ensure it is not constricting the cord or ilioinguinal nerve. The external oblique is closed with a 3-0 Vicryl in a continuous fashion. Care is taken to avoid injuring or trapping the ilioinguinal nerve. Marcaine with epinephrine is injected under the external oblique (without a needle). Scarpa's fascia is closed with 3-0 Vicryl followed by Camper's fascia in a continuous fashion. The subcutane-

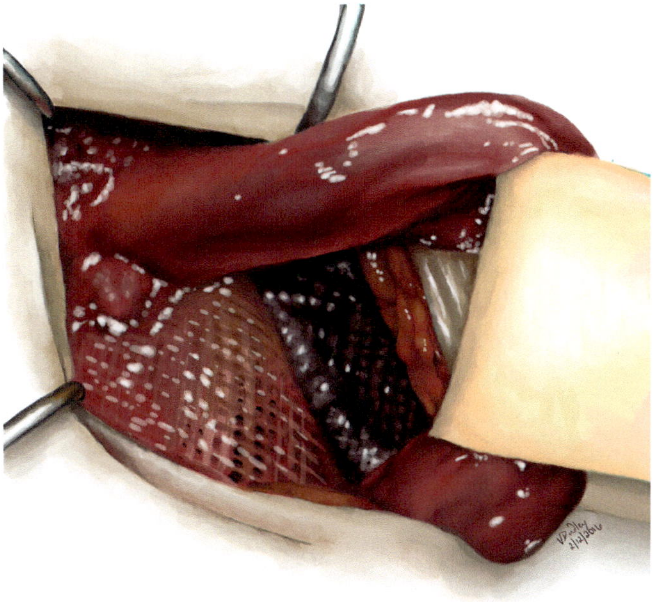

Fig. 14.5 A polyethylene patch is soaked in Betadine then placed on the floor of the inguinal canal with a 1.25 cm diameter pre-cut round opening for the spermatic cord to pass through. (From Schulster et al. [1]; with permission)

ous tissue is approximated with 4-0 monofilament in a horizontal mattress fashion. 0.25% Marcaine with epinephrine is injected into the subcutaneous tissue. The skin is closed with a 5-0 Monocryl in a subcutaneous fashion, the skin is reinforced with steri-strips and dressed.

The postoperative instructions provided to patients following inguinal hernia repair is the same as that for microsurgical varicocele repair, as described in Chap. 3.

14.2 Complications

By utilizing systemic antibiotics plus constant antibiotic solution irrigation, we have had no infections in any of our several hundred cases. We have had no cases of chronic (more than 3-month postoperatively) pain. There was one recurrent hernia.

Reference

1. Schulster ML, Cohn MR, Najari BB, Goldstein M. Microsurgically assisted inguinal hernia repair and simultaneous male fertility procedures: rationale, technique and outcomes. J Urol. 2017;198(5):1168–74. https://doi.org/10.1016/j.juro.2017.06.072. Epub 2017 Jun 19.

15 Final Thoughts

15.1 Thoughts on the Use of Robots in Male Fertility Surgery

Robots traditionally have been most useful in operations that require large incisions like radical prostatectomies and radical nephrectomies. A robot will allow you to do this laparoscopically, being able to perform the surgery by controlling the robot arm through a much smaller incision. All the surgery that I describe is done through very small incisions. The robot offers no advantage in terms of reducing the size of the incisions; in fact, it can make it more complicated to try and get the robot arm in the scrotum. The only thing it does is eliminate hand tremor, which can turn a poor surgeon into an adequate one. This is not a good enough reason to use a robot. Furthermore, it tremendously increases the cost of microsurgery.

15.2 "Goldsteinisms"

- Use detailed checklists specific to and prior to starting every surgery.
- If a resident, fellow, or medical student asks the attending surgeon "Why do you do something that way?" and the answer is "I've always done it that way," that is not an acceptable answer.
- Use two hands for every microstitch. Always have one hand supporting the other.
- Use a micro-bipolar for skin bleeders. It will not burn the skin.
- Transillumination of the cord with a properly positioned operating room light allows isolation of the vas with the vasal sheath enclosing it with minimal bleeding. It allows you to poke through the cord in an avascular spot.
- For doing a tension-free anastomosis or an orchiopexy for an undescended testis, get as much length as you think you need, and then get some more.
- Tie every knot square and flat for the rest of your life.
- Satisfaction with "good" is the enemy of perfection.
- Patience and persistence are among the keys to being a superb surgeon. Never give up!
- Place a heating pad on the scrotum to relax the dartos muscle prior to physical exam. This is more important than a scrotal ultrasound.
- If you encounter a difficult to find bleeder during the macro part of any operation, put pressure on it with a sponge and bring in the microscope. You will find it every time.
- If you want to be a fast surgeon, slow down and never make a mistake. Economy of motion is also key to being a good rock climber and to being a faster surgeon.
- Do the right thing; every time, all the time.
- *CANI*: Constant and never-ending improvement.
- My goal is not to train future microsurgeons that are as good as me; my goal is to train microsurgeons who are better than me.
- Do the kind thing and do it first. (Sir William Osler)
- Kindness is more powerful than cunning.
- Try to learn something about everything and everything about something. (Thomas Henry Huxley)
- For every complex problem there is a simple answer, and it is wrong! (H.L. Mencken)

15.3 Personalities of Surgeons and Fighter Jocks

Having been both, humility is not the trait that can be used to describe either. As Ed Dwight wrote in his 2009 autobiography, "Fighter pilots are universally Type-A personalities, independent, aggressive, daring, risk-oriented, total control freaks, and the real good ones are usually arrogant asses. Exercising absolute control over a complex … high-speed machine that requires the ultimate in training, superior intellectual input, and psychomotor reaction requires such a personality."

M. Goldstein, *Atlas of Male Infertility Microsurgery*, https://doi.org/10.1007/978-3-031-31601-2_15

15.4 Reflections of a PGY50 Surgeon

Surgical practice is among the most demanding, difficult, and unforgiving professions in the world. Kind and nice people are often the most successful. It is important to maintain your cool. Aequanimitas, as Sir William Osler said, is essential in the operating room. A cool, controlled approach is best when things get tough. "This game is for big people, and if you cannot take the heat in the kitchen, do not cook" [1].

Tell the truth, all the time, every time [2]. Be impeccable about your word.

Do not schedule surgery on the same day you have to travel. Never operate with the thought in your head that you must get out of the operating room by a certain time. Do not look at the clock when you operate.

Never bad-mouth another surgeon to a patient. Talk to that surgeon directly yourself. Never make assumptions, not about what a patient says another surgeon did, or even about what another surgeon says they saw or did. Find out for yourself.

References

1. Elsey J. Reflections on surgical practice: lessons learned along the way and notes to my young colleagues. J Am Coll Surg. 2021;233:639–43.
2. Farid H. Sanctity. JAMA. 2023;329(7):537–8.

Suggested Reading

Bean WB. Sir William Osler: aphorisms from his bedside teachings and writings. Br J Philos Sci. 1954;5(18):172.

Woods D. The quotable Osler. BMJ. 2003;326(7383):289.

Index

M. Goldstein, *Atlas of Male Infertility Microsurgery*, https://doi.org/10.1007/978-3-031-31601-2

GPSR Compliance

The European Union's (EU) General Product Safety Regulation (GPSR) is a set of rules that requires consumer products to be safe and our obligations to ensure this.

If you have any concerns about our products, you can contact us on ProductSafety@springernature.com

In case Publisher is established outside the EU, the EU authorized representative is:

Springer Nature Customer Service Center GmbH
Europaplatz 3
69115 Heidelberg, Germany

Batch number: 10731530

Printed by Printforce, the Netherlands